Orthopedic Practice Management

Eric C. Makhni • Melvin C. Makhni
Eric F. Swart • Charles A. Bush-Joseph
Editors

Orthopedic Practice Management

Strategies for Growth and Success

Springer

Editors
Eric C. Makhni
Department of Orthopedic Surgery
Henry Ford Hospital
Detroit, MI
USA

Eric F. Swart
Department of Orthopedic Surgery
UMass Memorial Health Care
Worcester, MA
USA

Melvin C. Makhni
Brigham and Women's Hospital
Harvard Medical School
Department of Orthopedic Surgery
Boston, MA
USA

Charles A. Bush-Joseph
Department of Orthopedic Surgery
Rush University Medical Center
Chicago, IL
USA

ISBN 978-3-319-96937-4 ISBN 978-3-319-96938-1 (eBook)
https://doi.org/10.1007/978-3-319-96938-1

Library of Congress Control Number: 2018962531

This Springer imprint is published by the registered company Springer Nature Switzerland AG
The registered company address is: Gewerbestrasse 11, 6330 Cham, Switzerland

Foreword

These are exciting times in medicine. Our health care delivery and payment systems are undergoing fundamental transformation from a system focused on the provision of health care services, to one that is focused on improvements in health. These changes create unique opportunities and challenges for orthopedic surgeons. In addition to being skilled technicians and excellent communicators, orthopedic surgeons entering practice today must be adept at using information about their outcomes and costs of delivering care in continuous performance improvement efforts; facile with ever growing and rapidly changing health information technology; and familiar with a variety of different contracting and integration strategies.

From understanding what type of practice environment is right for you, to learning effective strategies for building and growing a practice, to gaining insights into tools and technologies that can be used to measure and improve patient outcomes, and identifying and evaluating professional and leadership development activities outside of clinical practice, this book will serve as a valuable reference guide for young orthopedic surgeons as they enter practice.

Practicing orthopedic surgery is both a great privilege and a grave responsibility; I hope you will find the insights provided on the pages herein by those who have come before you to be helpful on your journey to what I am certain will be a long, productive, and rewarding career.

Austin, TX, USA
November 2017

Kevin J. Bozic, MD, MBA

Preface

One of the most common questions I get by my colleagues and residents is, "How do you use your MBA in your medical practice?" And of course, without fail, my only response is, "I use it all the time!" I was very fortunate to have had the opportunity to seamlessly pursue my Masters of Business Administration (MBA) during medical school. However, due to a variety of reasons, most of my colleagues did not have this opportunity.

While many may believe that a formal coursework is required to learn the "business" fundamentals of clinical orthopedics, our hope is that this book may serve as a useful guide and even alternative to that coursework. In fact, most of the best, business-savvy orthopedic surgeons I know never took a course in management, or finance, or marketing, and instead became proficient through self-education and trial-and-error. Moreover, most of what I "wish" I knew when I started my clinical practice was not taught in business school. So – for those of you who do not have an MBA – rest assured that you can be a pro in practice management without ever paying a dollar of tuition (except maybe, for this book and others!).

Our main goal in this book is to provide readers with a brief introduction to many of the fundamental aspects of practice management. While this is written from an orthopedic focus, our hope is that practitioners in other specialties may find useful information within the chapters ahead. On the other hand, we realize that it is impossible to cover every topic relevant to practice management in one book. Therefore, we hope that we can continue to publish and review this guide so that we not only stay current in the subject matter, but also continue to comprehensively cover all the salient topics that matter most to practitioners.

As you progress through the chapters of this book, please remember a few core principles. First, and foremost, this book is meant to be an introduction. There is a *wealth* of information out there that augments and enhances the text ahead. There are several resources from the business world that are very powerful to practicing orthopedics. For those of you who have daily commutes, I recommend you download any of the several management-oriented podcasts (most of them are free). Some of these include Career Tools, Manager Tools, and reviews from the *Harvard Business Review*. There is no shortage of helpful textbooks as well that you can similarly listen to in the car or train in audio-book format or in text/Kindle format as well. The ones that I have found most helpful have been those focused on effective management strategies as well as those focused on communication and leading teams. Make sure to explore the business section of your local bookstore (brick and mortar or online) to see what other books are out there that will help you become a successful practitioner.

Second, never forget that formal education is more accessible than ever. You do not have to find a 2-year break in your education or practice to go and pursue a formal MBA. There are numerous alternatives to such an education. Many business schools offer online curricula that can be completed on nights and weekends. Other schools – including the top schools in the country – offer "Executive Education" programs that can be focused on a specific subject matter or broad and inclusive of a typical (but condensed) MBA coursework. Finally, there are numerous non-MBA degrees that are tailored to professionals in healthcare. Examples include Master of Healthcare Administration, Master of Public Health, and many others.

Ultimately, you are reading these pages because you have an interest and desire to understand how the "nonclinical" world works. We thank you for taking the time to explore the contents of this book, and we welcome any and all feedback that you might have. Please feel free to reach out to us (orthopedicpracticemanagement@gmail.com) and share your thoughts and comments with us so that we can work to implement this feedback into future versions of the book.

West Bloomfield, MI, USA Eric C. Makhni

Contents

Contributors

Avinesh Agarwalla, BS Rush University Medical Center, Midwest Orthopedics at Rush, Chicago, IL, USA

Rush University Medical Center, Department of Orthopedic Surgery, Chicago, IL, USA

Stephen Bartol, MD, MBA, FRCSC CMO for Henry Ford Innovations, Henry Ford Health System, Department of Orthopedic Surgery, Detroit, MI, USA

Jacob Blanchett, BS Division of Sports Medicine, Department of Orthopedic Surgery, Henry Ford Health System, West Bloomfield, MI, USA

Peter Borowsky, BS Division of Sports Medicine, Department of Orthopedic Surgery, Henry Ford Health System, West Bloomfield, MI, USA

Kevin J. Bozic, MD, MBA Dell Medical School at The University of Texas at Austin, Department of Surgery and Perioperative Care, Austin, TX, USA

Charles A. Bush-Joseph, MD Department of Orthopedic Surgery, Rush University Medical Center, Chicago, IL, USA

Christopher J. Dy, MD, MPH Washington University School of Medicine, Department of Orthopedic Surgery, Division of Hand and Upper Extremity Surgery, Department of Surgery, Division of Public Health Sciences, St. Louis, MO, USA

Mohsin S. Fidai, MD Henry Ford Health System, Department of Orthopedic Surgery, Detroit, MI, USA

Brian Forsythe, MD Rush University Medical Center, Midwest Orthopedics at Rush, Chicago, IL, USA

Rush University Medical Center, Department of Orthopedic Surgery, Chicago, IL, USA

Nicholas B. Frisch, MD, MBA Ascension Crittenton Hospital, Rochester Hills, MI, USA

Edward Goldberg, MD Department of Orthopedic Surgery, Rush University Medical Center, Chicago, IL, USA

Kenneth R. Gundle, MD Orthopedic Oncology, Orgeon Health and Science University, Department of Orthopedics and Rehabilitation, Portland VA Medical Center, Operative Care Division, Portland, OR, USA

Fady Y. Hijji, MD Department of Orthopedic Surgery, Rush University Medical Center, Chicago, IL, USA

Toufic R. Jildeh, MD Henry Ford Health System, Department of Orthopedic Surgery, Detroit, MI, USA

Krishna T. Kudaravalli, BS Department of Orthopedic Surgery, Rush University Medical Center, Chicago, IL, USA

Ramin M. Lalezari, BA Washington University School of Medicine, Department of Orthopedic Surgery, St. Louis, MO, USA

Natalie L. Leong, MD Rush University Medical Center, Midwest Orthopedics at Rush, Chicago, IL, USA

Rush University Medical Center, Department of Orthopedic Surgery, Chicago, IL, USA

William N. Levine, MD New York Presbyterian/Columbia University Medical Center, Department of Orthopedic Surgery, New York, NY, USA

Vincent A. Lizzio, BS Wayne State University School of Medicine, Henry Ford Hospital, Department of Orthopedic Surgery, Detroit, MI, USA

Joseph M. Lombardi, MD Orthopedic Surgery, Columbia University Medical Center, Department of Orthopedic Surgery, New York, NY, USA

Joseph S. Lombardi, MD JFK Medical Center, Edison Surgical Center, Department of Orthopedic Surgery, Edison, NJ, USA

Eric C. Makhni, MD, MBA Division of Sports Medicine, Department of Orthopedic Surgery, Henry Ford Health System, West Bloomfield, MI, USA

Melvin C. Makhni, MD, MBA Brigham and Women's Hospital, Harvard Medical School, Department of Orthopedic Surgery, Boston, MA, USA

Michael J. McCaslin, CPA Somerset CPAs and Advisors, Indianapolis, IN, USA

Fabien Meta, BS Wayne State University School of Medicine, Henry Ford Hospital, Department of Orthopedic Surgery, Detroit, MI, USA

Daniel J. Miller, MD Gillette Children's Specialty Healthcare, St. Paul, MN, USA

Vasilios (Bill) Moutzouros, MD Division of Sports Medicine, Henry Ford Health System, Department of Orthopedic Surgery, Detroit, MI, USA

Hamadi A. Murphy, MD, MS The Rothman Institute at Thomas Jefferson University, Department of Orthopedic Surgery, Philadelphia, PA, USA

Ankur S. Narain, BA Department of Orthopedic Surgery, Rush University Medical Center, Chicago, IL, USA

Kyle Pilz, MMS, PA-C RUSH University Medical Center, Department of Sports Medicine, Midwest Orthopedics at RUSH, Chicago, IL, USA

Richard N. Puzzitiello, BS Rush University Medical Center, Midwest Orthopedics at Rush, Chicago, IL, USA

Rush University Medical Center, Department of Orthopedic Surgery, Chicago, IL, USA

Gregory D. Schroeder, MD The Rothman Institute at Thomas Jefferson University, Department of Orthopedic Surgery, Philadelphia, PA, USA

Arjun J. Sebastian, MD The Rothman Institute at Thomas Jefferson University, Department of Orthopedic Surgery, Philadelphia, PA, USA

Weilong J. Shi, MD The Rothman Institute at Thomas Jefferson University, Department of Orthopedic Surgery, Philadelphia, PA, USA

Kern Singh, MD Department of Orthopedic Surgery, Rush University Medical Center, Chicago, IL, USA

Christie Stawicki, BS The Rothman Institute at Thomas Jefferson University, Department of Orthopedic Surgery, Philadelphia, PA, USA

Sasha Stine, MS Wayne State University School of Medicine, Henry Ford Hospital, Department of Orthopedic Surgery, Detroit, MI, USA

Eric F. Swart, MD Department of Orthopedic Surgery, UMass Memorial Healthcare, Worcester, MA, USA

Joseph S. Tramer, MD Henry Ford Hospital, Department of Orthopedic Surgery, Detroit, MI, USA

Alexander R. Vaccaro, MD, PhD, MBA The Rothman Institute at Thomas Jefferson University, Department of Orthopedic Surgery, Philadelphia, PA, USA

Mike West, MBA, CPA The Rothman Institute at Thomas Jefferson University, Department of Orthopedic Surgery, Philadelphia, PA, USA

Kelly H. Yom, BA Department of Orthopedic Surgery, Rush University Medical Center, Chicago, IL, USA

Part I
Starting and Building a Practice

Chapter 1
What to Look For In a New Job Opportunity: Strategic, Personal, and Legal Considerations

Eric F. Swart

If This Is Your First Job

If this is the first time you are applying for a job outside of the standard training "pipeline" of college, medical school, and residency, there are a few crucial differences in this process that are worth considering.

First, as an attending orthopedic surgeon, **you have a *lot* of value**. You are highly trained, and will be billing and collecting hundreds of thousands (or millions) of dollars annually, and will generate profit for both your practice and the healthcare system you practice in. This will stand in stark contrast to what life has been like in training thus far, and one of the most common mistakes for young surgeons is to underestimate their own value and contributions.

Further, unlike medical school, residency, and fellowship, the search for a job *really is a two-way fit*. You are not one of hundreds of applicants applying for multiple training "spots," where most qualified applicants could satisfactorily accomplish the job requirements. You are looking to join a practice where your individual contributions will be significant, and you will be entering into a long-term, complex relationship with the group you join. The importance of understanding what you want out of that relationship from the group, and what the group expects out of that relationship from you is crucial.

Along those lines, *the job description for a practicing orthopedic surgeon is relatively flexible*. As opposed to the role of a junior resident which has very concrete and well-defined requirements and obligations, recognize that as a practicing physician you have significantly more control over how you spend your time and what you want to choose to focus on. This is an opportunity to define your professional life and center it around your personal priorities and interests.

E. F. Swart
Department of Orthopedic Surgery, UMass Memorial Healthcare, Worcester, MA, USA

E. C. Makhni et al. (eds.), *Orthopedic Practice Management*,
https://doi.org/10.1007/978-3-319-96938-1_1

Define What Matters to You

Before even communicating with any prospective employers, the first step in looking for a new job opportunity is to define what your personal and professional priorities are. This should be as explicit and formally stated as possible, in order to force concrete description and prioritization, which will make decision-making more straightforward at later stages.

One commonly utilized method is to start by listing all of the attributes that you will take into account when considering a potential position. At this stage, just list any factor that you think you will be considering. Do not worry about assigning value or importance yet. A potential list of factors might be:

- *Clinical Practice Type:* Private practice, academics, or something in between? You may want to consider and evaluate multiple different types of positions, but this is a core distinction you should consider early in the process.
- *Geography*: Where you are willing to live and practice plays a central role in this process. For some, this will be a primary factor, while for others it may be relatively flexible.
- *Salary/Reimbursement*: How much you are paid, and how that pay is structured are critical factors. Some may want a more reliable, guaranteed income, while others may be more interested in positions with higher potential pay but less income stability.
- *Mentorship Opportunities*: The availability of senior partners in the practice to act as mentors and provide guidance may be a crucial factor for some, especially those earlier in their careers. It is important to evaluate not only the presence of mentors, but their availability and interest in mentoring as well.
- *Research Potential*: Some applicants will make research a primary consideration, while others will have minimal interest in research. No matter what your situation, you should clearly identify the expectations and requirements for research in any potential position, and make sure it is compatible with your goals and interests.
- *Stability*: Is this a well-established position with multiple partners who have been present for many years, or is this a new/expanded position where the prospects for success are less reliable? How much recent turnover has there been in the practice, both at entry-level positions and leadership positions? The importance of stability of a position will be a function of your current life and family situation, and your short- and long-term goals.
- *Growth Potential*: Is there a clear path for growth and advancement within the practice? How dedicated is the group to your success? Are your personal goals aligned with their strategic growth plans?
- *Teaching Role*: Will you work with residents? Physician assistants or nurse practitioners? Virtually all positions have at least some teaching component, although the amount and importance of that component can be highly variable, and should match your level of interest.

- *Administrative Role*: What responsibilities will you have outside of clinical and academic duties? Are you interested in being involved in process and quality improvement, or financial management? Making sure your interests match with expectations is crucial.
- *Work-Life Balance*: Finally, what will your life be like outside work? How much flexibility is there, and how important is that to you? At different stages of life, people may have very different priorities about balance between work responsibilities and life outside the hospital. Even the best work environment can be unsustainable if there is not room for meaningful life outside of work.

Once you have thought through and defined the aspects of job opportunities that you will be considering, *define what matters most to you*. The simplest way to do this is to rank the factors you identified from "most important" to "least important." For some, geography and work-life balance will be their major considerations, while for others it may be salary and growth potential. *If you have family members centrally involved in your life, involve them heavily in this process*. Clearly identifying what is most important to you and your family will make decision-making less daunting when you are evaluating multiple opportunities by providing a structure through which to compare them, and by reminding you of what you have decided is the most important.

The Stages of a Job Search

The process of finding, applying for, and evaluating different job opportunities is more fluid and open-ended than most of the preceding stages of medical training (in medical school, residency, fellowship, etc.), which generally have clear, concrete timelines, and a set of well-defined steps required to obtain a position. In contrast, evaluating orthopedic positions is much more dynamic and flexible, so staying organized, being a clear communicator, and having a solid plan is essential. In general, the process can be broken down into a few stages:

- *Early Communication*: Prior to any formal communication about a specific position, contact with potential future employers occurs on a more informal basis. Word-of-mouth, referrals, and networking are crucial for identifying and staying in touch with potential future employers. Cast a broad net early by using academic meetings, courses, and other venues to make connections. Keep track of communications, as they often end with vague plans to retouch base in a set period of time when things may become more definite. Following up reliably is a way to demonstrate sustained interest and commitment, and show a potential employer that you are serious about taking the discussion further.
- *The Interview Process*: At some point, informal conversations will transition into plans to formally interview for a position. The interview process itself is highly variable, may involve multiple rounds, and sometimes even formal presentations. This is usually a "feeling out" process where you determine how closely your

interests match their needs, and if your skills and personality are a good fit for the group.

- *Negotiation*: In truth, the negotiation process starts the first time you contact a potential employer, but it typically becomes more formal and concrete during the interview process and in follow-up communication after the process. It is important during this process to have a strong position on what you can bring to the practice, and to know what your "asks" are. The clearer a sense you have at the onset of what your "musts" or "deal breakers" are vs. what your "wants" are, the more straightforward these conversations can be. An important negotiation principle is, whenever possible, to have a strong alternative available (sometimes described as Best Alternative to Negotiated Agreement, or BATNA). If this is your first job, it means trying to align the timeline so you are discussing multiple offers concurrently, to give you a direct basis for comparison and a stronger bargaining position. If you are already employed, it means understanding how any offer compares to your current position, and having a clear sense for what additional benefits it would take to get you to switch positions.
- *Finalization and Contract Signing*: Until you have a formal, written offer letter or a job contract, you do not have a job. See the section below about important details of the contract itself, but this phase is an important part of the process of transitioning the negotiation process above into an explicit, mutually agreed-upon plan. The more concrete you can be in terms of goals, objectives, deliverables, and requirements, the easier things will be in the future if there are any disagreements or concerns.

The Job Contract

The prospect of reading, interpreting, and negotiating over the fine legal details in a job contract can be harrowing to physicians, usually due to unfamiliarity with the terminology and a lack of formal training in both the meaning and the importance of several items commonly found in orthopedic contracts. However, in addition to verbally negotiating over the circumstances of a new job opportunity, it is critical that the contract also be carefully negotiated over to make sure it accurately reflects the position as defined by both groups. Below are some key tips and terms in the contract negotiation process:

- *Read the Contract!* This may seem obvious, but many surgeons never formally read through the contract themselves due to unfamiliarity with the terms and the misperception that the language in the contract will always reflect the content of the conversations that have happened. You should read the whole contract, in entirety, and understand precisely what you (and your employer) are agreeing to.

- Likewise, *if something is important to you about your job, make sure it is written down*. Prospective employers willing to verbally agree to conditions but unwilling to put it in writing should be a red flag in the negotiation process. In some circumstances (like many large academic centers), the formal employment contract is standardized, and you may be told that there is no room for negotiation of the contract language. If that is the case, you can still have a separate, formal written agreement between you and your employers about the things you are agreeing to outside of the standard physician contract.
- *If you are going to use a contract lawyer*: Having your contract reviewed by an attorney representing your interests is generally recommended under most circumstances. *Strongly consider using an attorney with specific experience in healthcare contracts*. Physician employment contracts have nuances and unique circumstances that not all attorneys may be familiar with. Make sure any attorney you use has the experience and skill set to best advocate for you. Additionally, *get them involved early*. If you plan on involving a lawyer of your own, tell your employer as early in the contract process as possible that you plan on doing so. If the contract has already undergone several rounds of negotiation and is in the finalization process, and then the process halts when an additional lawyer is brought in by you, it can be frustrating to your potential employer and sour negotiations.

Terms to be familiar with and specific items to look for in the contract:

- *Terms of contract and renewal terms*: Carefully examine the timing of the contract and renewal terms, to know how long the contract is valid for, and when it will be re-negotiated. Some contracts will renew automatically if both parties are happy, and others have conditions that necessarily expire after a certain time. Of note, pay attention to the termination conditions (see below). You may have a "3-year contract," but if either party can terminate without cause with a 90-day notice, it is effectively only a 3-month contract. This can affect the stability of your position and other personal life choices you may make.
- *Partnership conditions and buy-in options*: In private practices, you may have the option to buy-in to the practice after a certain period of time (typically about 3–5 years). Read this carefully to understand what the financial commitment for a buy-in requires, and what assets and revenue streams are associated with the practice.
- *Malpractice insurance and tail coverage*: The structure of malpractice coverage is generally one of two kinds:
  - *Claims Made*: Claims-made coverage means that you are covered by the policy only if the claim is made while you are in the practice.
  - *Occurrence*: Occurrence coverage means that you are covered as long as the issue involved the lawsuit happened while you were in the practice.

Practically, this means that occurrence is more desirable than claims made. For example, if you had a claims-made policy, then left the practice, and the next year were sued for a patient care event that happened while you were in the practice, you would not be covered by a strict claims-made policy. In that instance, coverage after you left the practice for incidents that occurred while in that practice must be purchased, which is called a "tail". The issue of who pays for the tail coverage in the event of contract termination can be essential (and expensive), and should be clearly delineated.

- *Restrictive Covenants*: Restrictive covenants broadly govern the ability of a physician to compete with a practice after leaving it. They take various forms including non-compete, non-solicitation, and confidentiality agreements. These are not permitted in some states, and the where they are allowed, the rules governing their application can be complex. If there is a restrictive covenant in the contract you are evaluating, this should be reviewed by your attorney to ensure your interests are protected, and that you understand what the consequences of leaving the group would be on your career and future practice.
- *Termination Conditions*: Be sure to understand the conditions for which either group can terminate the contract. The grounds for early termination can be "for cause" or "at will" (without a cause). If the contract can be terminated without cause, check what the repercussions of that termination mean: Do restrictive covenants still apply? Who will pay for the tails on malpractice insurance? Failure to closely evaluate this possibility can leave you financially and legally exposed if it is not clearly defined.

The Final Decision

Before making any final decisions, make sure to do due diligence and research the practice beyond the information they provide: Call former practice members who have recently left, get access to publicly available financial records, call members of other practices in the area to find out their reputation, and use whatever means you can to confirm (or change) the information you have available to make your decision.

Once you have gathered as much information as you can, go back to your original priorities, and explicitly work through how the new position will affect you (and your family). Remember that no job opportunity is ever perfect, but you can evaluate the important changes: Are you improving the areas that are important to you? Are there drawbacks or issues with the new opportunity areas where you are willing to sacrifice? By advocating for yourself during the negotiation process, gathering and corroborating detailed information about the practice, and evaluating the opportunity against your predefined list of priorities, you can maximize the chance that you will make the best decision and put yourself in a position for future success.

Recommended Reading

1. Grewal S. CareerMedicine.com's Mini Guide to thysician job search: CreateSpace Independent Publishing; Feb 2009.
2. Harbin T. The business side of medicine: what medical cchools don't teach you: Mill City Press; Dec 2012.
3. Higgins NB. Transition 2 practice: 21 things every doctor must know in contract negotiations and the job search: Two Harbors Press; Oct 2015.
4. Shaw K. The ultimate guide to finding the right job after residency. McGraw-Hill; Dec 2005.

Chapter 2
Partnership, Ancillaries, and Other Considerations

Michael J. McCaslin and Nicholas B. Frisch

Introduction

Healthcare is a continually changing environment, which impacts the formation and ongoing succession planning for an orthopedic group practice. Generational changes coupled with a dynamic healthcare environment create many challenges for orthopedic group practices. A succession plan is the structure which enables the addition of new physicians, facilitating the retirement and related buy-out of the senior physicians. Ultimately, appropriate succession planning leads to the continued growth and prosperity of the practice.

Understanding the importance of healthcare policy changes as well as the impact of generational shifts is critical to helping your practice successfully navigate forward. Partnership, income distribution formulas, buy-in and buy-out values and structures, and the viability of long-term practice successes are often intricately tied to policy and generational shifts. The passage of the Affordable Care Act (ACA) and the introduction of the Generation X (Gen X) and Millennials into the orthopedic group practice workforce have left a permanent impact on orthopedic group practice succession planning. The ACA pushed hospitals to become health systems, which resulted in hospitals hiring physicians across all specialties including primary care, cardiology, and orthopedics. Ultimately, there is great uncertainty today regarding the state of the ACA as new healthcare legislation continues to be debated among lawmakers. Data from the American Medical Association Physician Masterfile showed that in 2001, 47.5% of all surgeons were self-employed, but by 2009 that

M. J. McCaslin (✉)
Somerset CPAs and Advisors, Indianapolis, IN, USA
e-mail: mmccaslin@somersetcpas.com

N. B. Frisch
Ascension Crittenton Hospital, Rochester Hills, MI, USA
e-mail: nick@gafrisch.com

E. C. Makhni et al. (eds.), *Orthopedic Practice Management*,
https://doi.org/10.1007/978-3-319-96938-1_2

number decreased by 15.4% [1]. Between 2006 and 2011, there was a 32% increase in the number of surgeons employed full-time by hospitals.

Gen X and Millennials did not go into medicine necessarily dreaming of owning their own medical practice and all of the management and financial issues that accompany this. There remains little to no formal business or management training in traditional medical school education. The increasing desire for hospitals to recruit and support employed physicians offers an appealing option and alleviates much of the administrative burden associated with running a successful practice [2]. Add to this, that senior physicians have an incentive to consider hospital employment so private practice survival is at risk. While we are witnessing a shift from volume- to value-based reimbursement, senior physicians and often their existing practices are not necessarily geared toward profitability under these new payment models. Furthermore, future compensation is potentially at risk due to a number of factors including healthcare regulatory and reimbursement changes, plus increased competition with hospital-employed physicians.

Putting this all together, the path to partnership, buy-in and buy-out, ancillaries, and related practice entities has changed dramatically. We believe there is still great value to the private practice model and if set up correctly, an incredible opportunity for personal and professional growth with long-term financial sustainability. The theme in this environment is ease of practice entry, affordability, and proper exit strategy. Ease of entry and affordability is the current path to recruit and retain the current new generation of physicians. This chapter will address the current state and environment for these issues as we see it in 2018 and beyond.

Qualifications for Partnership/Partnership

There are many different legal structures in which a medical practice operates. This includes a Sub-Chapter C corporation, a Sub-Chapter S corporation, a Limited Liability Company (LLC), a Limited Liability Partnership (LLP), and a Partnership or a sole proprietorship (schedule C on the individual tax return). These different entities result in different names for the partners such as shareholder, partner, member, etc. We will reference all as "partners" for purposes of this discussion.

For a long period of time, the track to partnership inside the orthopedic private group practice industry had a pretty standard set of criteria which was utilized by most orthopedic group practices. We acknowledge that there are many variations on this model and it may not apply to every group. A newly recruited physician was required to work 2 years as an "Associate Physician," meet all Board Certification requirements (passing the written and oral Board requirements), and be in the black (producing net income when considering the Associate Physician's compensation) in terms of financial performance. Barring any personality or behavior issues, the Associate Physician was invited to become a partner, execute the buy-in in accordance with the buy-in formulas, and execute the appropriate legal documents.

Even with the competition of hospital employment, there are still a significant number of private practice groups and partnership opportunities for the orthopedic surgeon. Many groups have general unwritten guidelines as to what it takes to become a partner in a practice. Groups that have written guidelines generally have a list that is flexible due to the challenges in recruitment in the current environment (i.e., now competing with hospitals to hire orthopedic surgeons and not just competing with other orthopedic groups). It is advisable to obtain a clear list of qualifications for partnership in advance, which could include the following:

- Patient and bedside manner reputation
- In office and personal communication style and demeanor
- Fellow physician communication style and demeanor
- Board eligible and certified by the completion of the second year of employment
- Being in the black (producing net income) under the associate physician income distribution formula
- Regular attendance at group practice meetings, marketing functions, and social functions
- Adherence to medical records group practice documentation requirements
- Adherence to quality of care group practice required data submissions
- Adherence to group practice patient-reported outcome forms completed (HOOS JR, KOOS JR, SF-12, etc.)
- Adherence to group practice mandated number of patient satisfaction surveys completed
- Participation in group practice call coverage and emergency department group practice call coverage requirements (unless a special deal has been negotiated)
- Generally contributing in a positive way to the group practice culture

This represents a general list, and not all groups may have all items on their list or even have a list. Some of these criteria are objective, and some of these criteria are subjective. These criteria are the starting point for the group to consider whether to offer partnership. Typically, meeting these requirements does not guarantee partnership will be offered, but usually is a starting point for the partnership discussion. Group practices do not want to be boxed in in terms of having to offer partnership. If the group decides it is going to offer partnership to a physician and this is communicated to the physician, there is a substantial amount of work to be done by the physician and the group to address all the partnership issues. This includes legal requirements, buy-in issues related to what could be a number of medical practice–related entities, and a number of other related financial issues (loan guarantees).

The orthopedic group medical practice could have a number of entities that represent the overall interest of the practice. This could include the medical practice legal entity (where the professional services and ancillary services are rendered), a real estate entity or multiple real estate entities tied to the medical office buildings the group may own, a surgery center entity that houses an ambulatory surgery center owned by the group, or an entity holding the physicians partnership interest in the ambulatory surgery centers (ASC) owned by the group and another entity and potentially skilled nursing facilities. Each of these entities becomes a part of the partnership process and could be structured differently in each group. Knowing what your groups' entities are and how they are structured is a critical part of the decision-making process before formally entering any practice.

Medical Practice Entity

The Core Orthopedic Medical Practice

The medical practice entity is the core entity for the orthopedic group practice. This is where the professional services are delivered as well as any group practice ancillary services. The orthopedic group medical practice entity typically includes some combination of the following:

- Professional practices services
- Imaging: X-ray, magnetic resonance imaging (MRI) and computed tomography (CT)
- Physical therapy (PT) and/or occupational therapy (OT)
- Durable medical equipment (DME)
- Pharmacy

Other, less commonly available ancillary services include ambulatory surgery centers (ASC) and urgent care facilities. Additionally, some practices have the ability to perform a variety of other services that derive revenue which may include platelet-rich plasma (PRP) and stem cell injections. These are the exception rather than the rule and will not be discussed as part of this chapter.

These ancillary service lines represent potential revenue streams that a partner could buy-in to selectively, or gain access to as a whole upon reaching partner status in the group.

Inside the medical practice entity, the driver of the practice entity is the provision of physician's professional services. Generally, these services are supported by staff (medical/clinical, administrative/executive) and fixed assets (furniture, fixtures, and equipment) required to provide core professional services. When the patients arrive for the provision of services, at the time of service, the patient will make their co-payment and then the patient and the practice will wait for the processing of the insurance claim before billing the patient for the balance of the patient's payment obligation (amount owed by patient when the patient deductible has not been met). The medical practice entity bills for the physicians' services, the claim is processed, and the insurance company remits to the practice the contractual amount they are obligated to pay the practice based on the contract negotiated with the practice. This payment by the insurance company takes into account the co-payment and deductible obligation for each patient. This process results in the medical practice entity having an "accounts receivable" asset.

Accounts receivable at any point in time in the life cycle of the practice represents the claims that have not yet been processed by the insurance company and the outstanding balance payable by patients related to their co-payment and unmet deductible. As professional service fee accounts receivables are collected, they make their way through the income distribution formula of the orthopedic group practice. Each physician within the practice has their own identified accounts receivable, and the partners of the practice have their accounts receivable flow through to their compensation.

The physician who is not yet a partner but working toward partner status typically would not have a legal claim to the accounts receivable. They are an "Associate Physician" with a claim only to the base compensation and incentive compensation they would have negotiated as part of their Associate Physician Employment Agreement. This employed physician is typically on some type of guaranteed salary with a potential amount of incentive compensation that such incentive compensation will vary by group in terms of how the incentive compensation is determined.

Every orthopedic group practice that hires a new physician out of a residency or fellowship program takes the risk of whether the physician will work out and make their way to partnership. This risk could be related to work ethic, patient satisfaction, the group's satisfaction with the clinical expertise of the physician, or just personality match. If the employment relationship does not work to the point of leading to partnership status, then typically the physician and the practice part ways. At this point, the practice is left with the departed employed non-partner physician's accounts receivable and any remaining overhead issues, legal issues, or simply the cost to find a replacement physician.

An Associate Physician who does not become a partner generally does not have a legal claim to the accounts receivable they generated and walks away from it on departure. Because there is no legal claim on departure, if the physician is offered the opportunity to become a partner, the historical industry approach was receivables generated before the physician became a partner belong to the "partners" and the new physician partner must start over in the generation of their accounts receivable. This approach was in essence deemed part of the physician's medical practice buy-in. In some groups, the physician was required to write a check for a calculated amount of the estimated receivables to be collected on behalf of the new partner physician. This clearly creates a financial burden for the new partner and must be understood and negotiated prior to making any formal commitments. In other practices, the receivables buy-in was simply handled through a compensation reduction structure with such reduction occurring over a 12–24–36-month period. The result of this was the collection of the new partners "Associate-related receivables" and allocation to the partners either as they were collected or in some ratable amount over the number of months noted. The 12–24–36-month reduced salary approach made the accounts receivable buy-in much more affordable for the new partner physician as it spreads the compensation reduction impact over a longer period of time.

Historically, this did not set well with the non-partner or Associate physician as the receivables represented their personal production and work effort. On the other hand, they were receiving a salary during this time to compensate for their productivity and since those accounts receivable payments were generated during their employment, the time of collection may be deemed irrelevant. Increased pressure on recruiting, hiring, and gaining a long-term employment commitment from the new physicians has become a significant challenge for private orthopedic group practices. To maintain a competitive advantage in the market, private groups have largely eliminated any accounts receivable buy-in for new partners. This means no check written for the purchase and no reduced compensation structures.

It is equally important to outline what happens to accounts receivable when a partner transitions out of the practice. A partner departure from the practice after defined minimum years of service and under retirement as defined by the practice, termination due to permanent disability, death, and termination from the practice with proper notice, the partner will receive their balance of professional service accounts receivable as they are collected. This is typically treated as a payment of deferred compensation. A partner leaving under terms other than those defined would typically not receive any of their receivables upon departure.

The second part of the buy-in to becoming a partner inside the medical practice is the buy-in for the fixed assets of the practice or the book value of the practice. Orthopedic and medical group practices in general are not asset accumulating businesses or net worth accumulating businesses. Typically, the net book value of these assets is nominal. Still, many groups may use a stock or partnership unit buy-in equal to the net book value of the assets excluding the assets that represent ancillary services assets (if there is a separate ancillary services buy-in.) On a per partner basis, this value or buy-in could be an amount ranging from ten thousand dollars per partner up to as high as several hundred thousand dollars per partner. Many groups have decided to eliminate annual calculations of book value and use a stated or fixed value for net asset or book value component of the buy-in. This might have some relevance to historical buy-ins but it is generally utilized to simply solicit a financial commitment from the new partner (i.e., requiring the new physician have some skin in the game).

It is important to note the stated value or fixed value buy-in will usually not be represented by assets on the books to support this value or buy-in amount. This is more representative of the group practice looking for the physician to make an investment that really will be treated more like a deposit for when the physician retires they will receive their deposit or buy-in amount back. If a private orthopedic group practice merges or joins another group practice as part of a merger strategy, it is very likely that the proceeds on selling the assets to the new entity joined or liquidating the assets will result in each physician receiving less than the stated dollar value amount in return. This value differential from merged value and stated value can be made up with additional deferred compensation to represent the difference in value. The funding of buy-outs over time is generally handled with the proceeds from the buy-in of new partner physicians. With a reasonable amount of planning, the timing is such that the money received by the practice for new partners is turned around and paid to the departing partners and thus the issue of asset values supporting the buy-in or buy-out is rarely an issue.

If an orthopedic practice prefers a book value approach to the partner stock buy-in, then a formula similar to the following is often utilized:

"Modified Book Value" shall mean the net equity of the company at the end of the company's calendar year, computed in accordance with accounting principles as consistently applied by the company, subject to the following:

- Modified Book Value shall not include any proceeds collected or collectible by the Company under any policy or policies of life or disability insurance insuring the life or disability of a member, as the result of death or disability of a member.
- Modified Book Value shall not include non-qualified deferred compensation assets or non-qualified deferred compensation liabilities.
- No additional allowance of any kind shall be made for the goodwill, trade names, or any other intangible asset or assets of the Company other than the aggregate dollar amount of any of those such intangible assets appearing on the most recent balance sheet of the Company prior to the determination of Modified Book Value.
- All retirement plan contributions payable and notes payable of the Company (including, without limitation, all purchase price obligations to previously departed partners, but excluding purchase price obligations to the departing partner) shall be included.
- Unpaid physician compensation, current year undistributed profits, prior year undistributed profits, and bonuses shall be accrued as a liability.
- Patient/insurance and ancillary accounts receivable shall be disregarded.
- Trade accounts payable shall be disregarded.
- All furniture, fixtures, and equipment will be adjusted to ensure that no asset shall be depreciated below 15% of original cost.
- The total of all medical and office supplies expense at the valuation date shall be divided by 12 and multiplied by 2 to account for 2 months of medical and office supplies on hand.
- All capitalized assets and related depreciation and debt related to PT, MRI, or other ancillaries as added by the practice from time to time shall be excluded from the Modified Book Value computation.
- The Modified Book Value shall be divided by the total number of shares to arrive at the Modified Book Value per share. To the extent the Modified Book Value per share multiplied by the number of shares needed to create an equal partnership interest is less than $25,000, then the total price for an equal interest in the Company for the share buy-in shall be $25,000. To the extent the Modified Book Value per share multiplied by the number of shares needed to create an equal partnership interest is greater than $25,000, then the total price for an equal interest in the company of the share buy-in shall be the Modified Book Value per share multiplied by the number of shares to be purchased.

Ancillary Services

The ancillary services of the practice could represent separate elements of buy-in and buy-out. X-ray services are typically incorporated with the core services of the practice so the ancillaries that could be looked at as having separate buy-in and buy-outs would be as follows:

- Advanced Imaging: magnetic resonance imaging (MRI) and computed tomography (CT)
- Physical therapy (PT) and/or occupational therapy (OT)
- Durable medical equipment (DME)
- Pharmacy
- Ambulatory Surgery Center (ASC) – usually in a separate legal entity but not always
- Urgent care

The change from percentage of billed charges of physician reimbursement for professional services to RBRVS instituted by Medicare in the early 1900s (and predominantly adopted by commercial payers over time) led to a dramatic change in the ancillary services performed in a private orthopedic group practice. Prior to the RBRVS system being implemented, an orthopedic practice was dominated by professional services rendered. Orthopedic physicians were compensated reasonably for their professional services under the percent of billed charges. Subsequent to this change to the RBRVS payment methodology by Medicare and the related reduction in professional services reimbursement, private orthopedic practices began adding ancillary services as an offset to the reductions in professional services reimbursement. In addition to the income generated from these services, the private orthopedic group practice discovered significant patient efficiencies and cost management benefits with all services housed in the location the patient received their primary orthopedic care. Thus, patients were not required to travel to multiple locations to receive each of these (MRI and PT/OT, to name a few). In addition, the private orthopedic group practice charges/fees for these services were generally less than the alternative providers for these services (MRI entities, PT entities, hospitals, etc.). Lastly, the orthopedic surgeon could better manage patient outcomes with these services housed inside the orthopedic practice.

To establish the ancillary services, there is some initial financial risk related to the acquisition of the equipment (MRI unit, physical therapy equipment, and machines), space build out to accommodate the new services, plus the additional rent expenses associated with the space expansion required to house the ancillaries and investments in new people. These start-up requirements and related debt generally placed the practice and the physicians in a financial risk position. There would likely be start-up losses funded by either personally guaranteed bank loans or reductions in compensation. Ultimately, the ancillary services generated significant income, so the private orthopedic group practice is left to address how a new partner will buy-in to the ancillary services net income stream.

While each of these ancillary services is supported by physical assets, they are primarily revenue and net income generating ancillaries. The value is not in the assets that support the ancillaries, but is in the nonphysician providers services rendered to the patients that generate the net income. These new service lines with initial start-up financial risk, orthopedics groups were challenged on how to approach the buy-in aspects for these ancillaries. Initially, the assets were included in the book value calculation for the purchase of partnership interest of the practice. However, since the ancillaries are revenue and income generating focused, most of the ancillary buy-ins have been converted to a form or function of the net income generated by the ancillaries.

In the early years of ancillaries and before the implementation of the Accountable Care Act, the ancillary buy-ins could be as high as three times earnings. The primary approach for this buy-in was a foregone income approach, whereby a physician would use a stair-step approach to access to a full partner share of ancillary net income. The new partner physicians with a three times multiple of ancillary net income buy-in could forego 100% of a full share of ancillary services net income for 3 years or could forego 50% of a full share of ancillary services net income for 6 years (50% × 6 years equals a three times earnings buy-in). The buy-out for the ancillary services net income stream would be mirrored on departure with the physician staying in the income stream for 3 years to produce a three times multiple on buy-out. With the pressure on recruitment of orthopedic physicians to private practice groups, most ancillary services buy-ins have been modified to a range of 6 months to 12 months of foregone income at varying percentages at varying percentages of annual net income to achieve the desired multiple.

On a partner departure from the practice after a defined minimum years of service and under retirement as defined by the practice, termination due to permanent disability, death, and termination from the practice with proper notice, the partner buy-out for ancillary services will mirror the buy-in. If there was a one-time multiple of income buy-in, then the departing partner physicians would receive 1 year of ancillary services net income after his/her departure. This would be paid monthly as the ancillary services net income was generated and paid to then practice partners. If ancillary net income were paid quarterly to the physician partners, then a departed partner would receive their ancillary services net income quarterly. These ancillary services payments to departed partners are typically treated as a payment of ancillary services deferred compensation.

The structuring of any partner buy-in or buy-out has tax implications to the partner buying in, the recipients of the buy-in, the partners who are being bought out, and the partners who are responsible for funding the buy-out of a partner. The foregone income approach on the ancillary services buy-in for a new partner allows the new partner physician to buy-in with pre-tax dollars. That is, the new partner physician does not have to go to the bank and borrow money for the ancillary net income buy-in and use after-tax compensation dollars to repay the bank loan. The new partner simply takes a reduction in taxable compensation as they take less of the ancillary services net income (taxed as compensation and ordinary net income). This foregone income approach for existing partners is not a tax advantage approach as the foregone income they receive from the new partner is taxed as ordinary income as they receive the new partner's share of the foregone ancillary services net income. If the new partner had to buy-in with a check upfront, which would be considered part of the stock purchase or unit purchase, these buy-in proceeds allocated to the existing partners would likely receive capital gains treatment that could be 15 points less than the ordinary income tax rates (difference between the highest ordinary income federal tax rate of 37% and capital gains tax rate of 25%).

While on the buy-in side, the existing partners have the adverse tax impact and the new partner the tax advantage impact, on buy-out, the gate swings the other way. The partners remaining behind receive the benefit of the payments to the departed physicians as being completely tax deductible, since they are paid as deferred compensation. If the payments were structured as a stock redemption, the payments would not be tax deductible and thus the practice would need to collect approximately 2 dollars for every dollar to be paid out. This would realistically result in reductions in compensation to the partner left behind. For the departed physician, the payments received as accounts receivable deferred compensation and ancillary services deferred compensation are taxed to the receiving partner as ordinary income and are tax deductible to the group. Therefore, the group avoids the need to collect to 2 dollars for every dollar paid out since the deferred compensation payments are 100% tax deductible. The partner receiving the payments does not receive the benefit of capital gains tax rates and is thus taxed as ordinary income rates on their deferred compensation payments.

Many private orthopedic group practices ancillaries are Designated Health Services (DHS) governed by the Stark Regulations or also referenced as the "self-referral" regulations. The governments concern (as pressured by those who lost these services when physician group practices decided to bring these services inside the group practice and pressured by the cost to the Medicare program) is an inappropriate economic incentive for the physicians who refer to services they own. This chapter will not go into the regulations themselves but rather address the risk each private orthopedic group practices faces. There have been numerous times over the years since the Stark Regulations were instituted where the government and lawmakers have threatened to outlaw the partnership owning these ancillaries (those which are DHS such as MRI, PT/OT, and DME) inside the private physician group practice. This risk has impacted how ancillary buy-ins and buy-outs have been structured. Utilizing a foregone income approach on the buy-in side over some number of months or years eliminates the risk for the new partner physician of taking out a loan and making an upfront payment for their ancillary buy-in. This risk is the new partner makes the upfront payment and suddenly the ancillary services are outlawed, the practice must divest, and the new physician loses the income stream they were counting on to help repay the loan. Under the foregone income approach, if the ancillary income stream goes away, the physician simply no longer has foregone income going to the other partner physicians.

The same issue or risk exists on the buy-out side. If the practice makes an upfront payment for the entire value to the departing partner, the risk exists that the ancillary income source is outlawed by the government. In the event, it is outlawed the physicians left behind need to repay the money paid upfront to the departed physician (typically funded with a bank loan) but have lost that income source which was expected to repay the loan. Thus, the buy-in and buy-out approach protects all parties.

Conditions on Buy-Out

Many private orthopedic group practices incorporate notification of intent to terminate employment requirements as a part of the buy-out economics. The practicing orthopedic physician is helping the practice service patient needs and helping to cover their share of the overhead of the practice. If that physician leaves without being replaced, the remaining physicians will possibly have to increase their workload to help cover the patient demand previously serviced by the departed physician. In addition, the overhead will not change upon the departure of the physician, so without a new physician to help pay for this overhead the remaining physicians will see an increase in overhead on a per-physician basis. Because of this risk, many practices will implement a time line for notification of intent to leave the practice and economic consequences on the buy-out tied to the timeline. For example, in order to receive the full value (100%) all of the buy-out elements, a physician may need to provide 18 months' notice of intent to terminate. If the physician provides less than 18 months' notice but more than 12 months' notice of intent to terminate, they would be eligible for 50% of the value of their buy-out and if the physician provides less than 12 months' notice of intent to terminate, the physician may receive no buy-out. Eighteen months' notice is the magic number as this is the standard time frame for being able to recruit a new physician.

Medical Real Estate Entity

Many private orthopedic group practices own the medical office building or multiple buildings, which house their office operations. This can be a significant asset that is completely tied to the success of orthopedic practice. Successful succession planning for the real estate entity housing these building requires a mandatory buy-in by new partners of the medical practice entity.

The primary challenges with a real estate investment for a medical practice are as follows:

- Managing the debt level on the building, understanding that most physicians are debt adverse.
- Managing the partnership so that you ensure all of the physicians are partners.

- Ensuring that all physicians can be equal partners or at least benefit from the annual lease payments which are expensed to all of the physicians through the group practice's income distribution formula.
- Managing the dollar value of the buy-in for physicians understanding the competition for recruiting physicians and the new physicians desire for manageable buy-in obligations.
- Accepting that partnership accrues with being a partner of the medical practice entity (which is paying the rent and impacting physician compensation), there must be the opportunity to buy-in. Once partnership with the medical practice ceases, then partnership in the medical practice–related assets should also cease.
- Determining how the building will be valued as part of the valuation of the interest for a new partner and a departing partner.
- Managing future buy-outs and related cash outflow to ensure there is a manageable impact on annual cash returns for the remaining physicians.
- Avoiding having a sale of the building be the only exit strategy for partners and potentially depriving the young physicians of their opportunity for partnership.

Private medical practice owned real estate in and of itself is not a commercial real estate investment or multi-tenant mixed-use real estate investment. Assuming the building is designed specifically to accommodate your practice, the success of this real estate venture is tied 100% to the success of the medical practice enterprise. Solutions for the buy-in and buy-out for the medical real estate require a balanced thought process that takes all physicians into consideration. We do note that in some cases there are multi-tenant mixed-use real estate investments but those are outside of the scope of this discussion.

A second significant point about closely held real estate is that the real estate entity always has a debt obligation. This obligation is either a mortgage obligation to a financial institution or if the building has no debt, then there is an obligation to pay all of the partners for the value of the building (i.e., a buy-out obligation). By way of example, a $10 million building with a $10 million mortgage owes the bank $10 million dollars. If that same $10 million building had no bank debt, then the partners are owed $10 million dollars in value on buy-out when they leave (their proportionate share of the $10 million dollars assuming a cost basis value for the building). Succession planning for a medical group includes succession planning for the medical group and all related entities. If all entities are not linked, those entities whose succession is not tied to the medical practice entity could be at risk to find a buyer who will offer reasonable value. We always recommend that private practice orthopedic groups mandate participation (partnership) in all entities upon becoming a partner physician in the medical group, which includes the medical office building real estate entity.

The first challenge a private practice orthopedic group faces with their medical real estate is how they are going to value the real estate for buy-in and buy-out purposes. Real estate values are historically tied to independent appraisals. However, the variation year over year in the results of those appraisals frustrates many physicians. Real estate appraisers determine the value of medical real estate using a comparable sales approach on a sale per square foot, a capitalization of net operating income approach, and a replacement cost approach. When these three different methodologies are completed, the appraiser most often relies on the capitalization of net operating income for determining value. Essentially, the cash flow generated by the lease payment from the medical practice entity to the real estate entity is what is most important in the marketplace. Net operating income is essentially the net income of the entity plus adding back depreciation and interest expense. The remaining expenses beyond depreciation and interest expense are nominal so some often reference capitalizing the rent income. This net operating income is divided by a market capitalization rate (6.5%, 7.0%, 7.5%, 8.0%, etc.) to determine the gross value of the building. From this gross value, the debt or mortgage on the building is deducted to arrive at the net value of the building. The following (Table 2.1) is a sample calculation which reflects the impact on value of the capitalization rate used by the appraiser (or in the event of a sale the buyer) of a medical office building:

The frustration for the physicians arises when the capitalization rate changes for the annual valuations each time a physician presents for buy-in or buy-out.

The first task for the private practice orthopedic group is to decide how they will value their building or buildings. The options are as follows:

- Original cost excluding annual depreciation. Very conservative approach which keeps the value of the building the same as when it was constructed. This is a predictable value year over year and growth in the net value occurs only as the mortgage balance is reduced.
- Annual appraisals from an independent appraiser. The issues with this approach have been discussed. There is an annual cost for the appraisal and the unpredictability on the value.
- Internal calculation of value using the capitalization of net operating income approach but select a conservative capitalization rate (see 8.0% above) and lock this rate into the legal documents so it is agreed this rate will be used for all valuations related to buy-in or buy-out transactions. This allows for growth in value as rent income grows by the escalator in place (i.e., cost of living adjustment) yet also creates a predictable valuation and eliminates the capitalization rate changes that show up in independent appraiser valuation approaches.

Once the valuation approach has been agreed upon, the next is an ever-increasing buy-in dollar amount that many new physicians just starting their practice may find cost prohibitive. As has been noted, private practice orthopedic groups are currently in one of the most difficult recruitment periods for orthopedic surgeons. This demand

Table 2.1 Sample capitalization rate table

Net operating income	$750,000.00	$750,000.00	$750,000.00	$750,000.00
Capitalization rate	6.5%	7.0%	7.5%	8.0%
Gross value	$11,538,461.54	$10,714,285.71	$10,000,000.00	$9,375,000.00
Mortgage	$(3,000,000.00)	$(3,000,000.00)	$(3,000,000.00)	$(3,000,000.00)
Net value	$8,538,461.54	$7,714,285.71	$7,000,000.00	$6,375,000.00

in excess of supply places significant control in the hands of the new physicians who are looking for a minimal outlay to buy into groups with maximum income opportunities. Without new physicians continually joining as partners, there is some risk to current partners with respect to having their buy-outs funded (or their building purchased).

If you cannot recruit new physicians, ultimately you will not have anyone to lease the buildings you own. As the value increases over time, the partners of the real estate entity will need to decide if there is a ceiling on the buy-in dollar amount that they would consider in order to keep the cost from being a deterrent to new partners. If the value grows to the point of not being affordable, then there are some additional formulas or procedures to address this affordability issue without the current partners losing equity/value in their investment.

There are several options and suggestions for structuring the buy-in to allow new partners to join. There is no perfect answer and there are positives and negatives with each approach. There is also no industry standard in terms of being able to say most groups handle this in a certain way. Each solution for a private practice orthopedic group is not necessarily a standalone approach as elements of each approach can be mixed and matched with other elements.

Real Estate Buy-In and Buy-Out Affordability Options

Option 1: Refinance

Each time a new partner is approved for partnership, the entity would go to a financial institution and borrow money at the highest loan to value ratio the bank is willing to loan. We would expect this would be 80 to 90% of the value under historical market conditions, but more likely 60 to 70% under current conditions (i.e., real estate market crash November 2008). The entity would then distribute all of the loan proceeds to the current partner(s) which in essence pays the current partners for the 60/70/80/90% of value that the entity was able to borrow. When the loan (or increase in loan amount) is recorded on the books and the proceeds disbursed to the then current partners, the net value of the entity will decrease by the loan amount and now we have lowered the buy-in required of the other physicians. An equal partnership interest would then be offered to the new partner based on a value determined (cost basis or using the agreed upon capitalization of net operating income as agreed upon by the physicians) now taking the new debt into account. The rent that will make its way to the current partners would go to service a higher level of debt which will cause some reduction in annual distributions. There may or may not be a lesser amount left for cash flow (i.e., distributions) depending on the terms of the financing (interest rate and length of the mortgage amortization such as 10 years versus 20 years). This approach avoids large personal loans taken out by the new partner purchasing an interest (the need for the new partner to go to the bank and borrow money to fund their buy-in), and puts the loan in the entity which owns the real estate.

This approach allows the entity to drive the buy-in cash value of the entity down to the desired level (which will be optimal for new recruits). The additional money borrowed would be distributed to the existing partners prior to the admission of a new partner (allowing them to receive their equity/value), which in turn serves the purpose of managing the total dollars to be paid on buy-in. The downside to this approach is the entity never reduces its institutional debt and everyone understands that there are times when having a lot of institutional debt limits one's flexibility. Additionally, you are at the mercy of the financial institution, as well as current market conditions and interest rates at the time of the refinance, which could add substantial interest costs, loan to value problems, or prepayment penalties with which to contend. As many witnessed during the post-2008 economic difficulties, limiting debt is one of the best ways to deal with difficult economic times that could affect your cash flow. An additional negative to this approach is related to any real estate growth strategies a private practice orthopedic group may be planning to execute. If the group is planning on using the equity in their current buildings to facilitate financing of new properties, this approach eliminates that equity and eliminates this tool as a growth option. It will force the group's growth strategy to count on cash contributions from the physicians.

Option 2: Become the Bank

Sell an equal interest at full value to the purchasing physician, but have the real estate entity take a note from the purchasing physician (i.e., new physician owes the real estate entity the money for their buy-in). All distributions from the real estate entity to the new physician would be withheld to account for interest and principal payments on this loan made by the entity to the new physician partner. The physician would only begin receiving distributions once the note to purchase the partnership interest was paid in full. If you set the note obligation to be paid off over a fixed term (i.e., 10 years), the physician may be required to use personal funds to make up the shortfall if the cash distributions from the real estate entity are not enough to cover the note. This approach does not eliminate concerns with respect to the total dollar amount of the buy-in, but does limit the immediate cash outlay to the purchasing physician. You could certainly require some cash outlay (i.e., an initial cash payment of $50,000) and issue a note for the balance from the purchasing physician. This cash investment ensures the new physician has some skin in the game. While this does introduce a cash concern on top of a valuation concern, it is not unreasonable to require some cash contribution by the new partner. This approach will also likely result in the new physician partner having phantom income as the rent payments will produce taxable net income to the new partner, but since the new partner will have their distributions applied to their buy-in note, they likely will not receive any cash distributions (or if they do it will likely be minimal distributions) to cover their tax liability on the net income generated and allocated to the new partner.

The second part of this internal financing approach is to distribute the cash paid in by each new partner to the existing partner in proportion to their ownership percentage. The balance of their equity required to get their equity down to the new equal level will be reflected in a note payable by the entity to each of these existing partners. All the distributions withheld from the new partners to pay their note obligations will in turn be distributed to the existing partners. In essence, the notes receivable the entity shows as being due from the new partner is matched in total dollars by the notes payable by the entity to the existing physician partners needed to buy down their ownership interest. These partners will also receive their share of the annual distributions. So for some period of time the existing partners still receive most of the cash distribution representing distribution of income and buying down of their ownership interest. The new physician partners are seeing an increase in their equity every year, just not an increase in cash distributions.

Typically, the interest rate on the note due from the new partner is either that published by the IRS, which is the lowest amount allowed to be charged, or a rate equal to the prime rate of interest on debt the practice has or the real estate entity.

The first and foremost goal is to get new physician partners in the medical real estate entity and establish a down payment on the new partners purchase of the interest at the level that the physicians generally feel is the break point on affordability. This is generally somewhere between $25,000 and $100,000 depending on the valuation of the entity and current partner structure. While this is a broad range, some of this will be impacted by the market and related cost of living.

The note payable by the new physician partner would be the equal value for an ownership interest in the real estate per physician less this down payment. The note payable to the existing physicians would be their equal value, less the cash down payment from the new physician partner if there is a distribution of this cash down payment. This approach does enable the existing physicians to maintain their existing cash flow from the investment because the new physician is receiving limited to no distributions as those are applied to service his or her buy-in. Thus, this cash is redistributed to the pre-existing partners.

The primary negatives to this approach are the amount of the buy-in obligation (even if represented by a note) and no cash flow from the investment and likely negative cash flow when debt service and tax payments are considered.

Option 3: Sell Partial Interest Each Year

Instead of borrowing from a bank, as in Option 1 or acting as the bank in Option 2, simply sell a partial partnership interest each year until the new physician partner owns an equal interest. The partial interest sold each year would either be at a predetermined level defined in the entity's legal documents, or at some other level ultimately to be determined by what the new physician partner could afford.

The primary issues with this approach are the total dollar amount of the purchase required to be an equal partner, and the fact the physician would not be an equal partner immediately, but instead may be several years away from being an equal partner. Based on the valuation approach chosen, it could take a considerable number of years for a new physician partner to be an equal partner. One other issue is the value will change each year (increase each year) with annual rent increases (if a capitalization of net operating income approach is used) and debt reduction (no matter which valuation approach is used), so the new partner will be paying more per unit each year of the buy-in. This scenario has the new partner chasing a moving finish line because the value grows each year adding to the buy-in burden required to ultimately achieve equal partnership status.

Option 4: Use of Member Months

Under a Members Months approach, the real estate entity takes the position that it is not important for new physician partners to purchase historical value that has been built up. Rather the new physician partner pays a par value amount (i.e., $50,000 as used in option 3 above) to buy-in and receive this par value amount when they leave, but they hold an interest in a future liquidity event based on the number of months ownership relative to all other partners number of months ownership accumulated. The rights to the future liquidity event are earned based on the number of months of partnership ownership. Step one of the process is all physicians buy-in for the “par” or “stated” value. We can use $50,000 by way of example. Then during their life as a partner and employee of the real estate entity and the private practice orthopedic group entity, they receive credit (tracked off books in an Excel spreadsheet) for each month they own the building. When they terminate, the terminated partner is paid their “par” or “stated” value of $50,000 and they sit holding their member months (no future distributions are available once a partner sells for your par value) to use for their claim for proceeds for a liquidity event. Thus if the building sold 10 years (or later) after they retired, they would participate in the net sale proceeds based on their member months divided by all physicians member months. During the 10 years (or more) in which they are waiting for the liquidity event, other physician partners are gathering member months so there is a dilution in equity (based on member months) but there should be an increase in value just based on debt reduction alone. All partners during partnership receive the same distribution so there are no distributions tied to longer term partnership and participation in the increase in value over the years.

The primary advantages of this model are as follows:

- The enterprise does not have to worry about funding buy-outs (other than par/stated value) for departing physicians.
- There are no market-based formulas (even if defined in the operating agreement) driving valuations, but rather all partners participate in the sale price as is actually

determined from the sale of the building and all buy-ins are at the same "par value."

- Long-term shareholders of the medical practice who have not been partners of the real estate will feel the equal distributions are justified, based on all of the months they paid the rent on the practice side, in spite of not being partners on the real estate side.

The disadvantages to this model are as follows:

- There is no annual recognition and return for the value created by those physicians who have owned the building longer and paid rent (an expense in the income distribution formula to the physicians on the medical practice side which such rent has funded the building) so no recognition of the equity created.
- Those physicians with built up equity will argue (with some justification) that equal distributions do not properly reflect return on cash invested or return on equity built up.
- The investment is illiquid as each physician is tied to the "liquidity" event so there could be long time (if ever) the departed partner ever sees the full value for the real estate.
- The real estate entity could feel pressure from a block of departed physicians to sell the building (even though they lose their voting interest on departure) because they want their cash when the younger physicians still want to own the building and build something of value for themselves.

Option 5: Use of Equity Notes

If the value grows to the point of not being affordable (assuming we are not using member months of partnership approach), there are some additional formulas and procedures to address this valuation issue, without the current partners or founding partners losing value or equity in their investment. These extra procedures include the determination of minimum dollars expected on buy-in, plus the use of equity notes as follows:

When the founding partners' equity positions exceed $50,000 (or some other agreed upon predetermined level), convert the existing equity greater than the targeted amount to debt for all current members so that each member is left with some small amount of equity. In essence rather than refinancing with a bank, the real estate entity performs an internal refinance by allocating the equity or value in excess of the threshold amount (i.e., $50,000) to notes payable to the current or founding partners.

This would leave the new buy-in amount for a new physician partner at $50,000 per partner for an equal partnership interest. This number is a *minimum* per partner purchase price, but at the time of the initial buy-in, a new partner could elect to buy-in up to the equalized value if they so desired at that time because they see a great return (cash distributions) on the investment. Over time as the current partner's equity increases, any equity amount over $50,000 would be converted to an equity note payable and moved to the liability section of the balance sheet, just like a bank finance mortgage note. As stated this is similar to a refinance with the bank, but uses the existing partners as the bank. Why pay interest to the bank on a refinance (Option 1) when you can pay it to the existing partners?

- The notes payable would pay quarterly interest at the 10-year Treasury note rate as established on January 1 of each year (or some other rate to be established by the physicians such as prime plus 2 points), and such rate shall be applicable for the entire year. Each January 1 the interest rate for the next calendar year shall be re-established based upon the Treasury note rate in effect each January 1.
- The note obligation can be set up to have excess cash flow pay down the debt on an annual basis or could be set up to only be payable upon termination from the real estate entity, and the corresponding termination from the private practice orthopedic group entity. All payments upon termination shall be in accordance with the provisions of the partnership agreement. Thus, it is not a demand note where a member can demand immediate payment. Generally, we see somewhere between 60 months (5 years) or 120 months (10 years) for buy-out notes from real estate entities. If the notes are paid down on an annual basis, the pay down of the equity for physicians with notes results in a redistribution of equity to the then partners.

It is important to reiterate a couple of key points if this option is utilized (convert equity to debt for existing partners). The current partners will still get their value. The value is simply structured as a note and equity. The entity is still obligated to purchase the interest of departing partners with that equity interest being the combination of the equity to debt note being combined with the equity ($50,000) on termination and the combination of the equity note, and equity rolled into a new note. While new partners will pay less for an equal partnership interest, the issuance of the notes and the payment of quarterly interest expense will lessen the net income available for distribution. Therefore, while they pay less to become a partner, they will receive less in annual distributions because there will be less in net income. In addition, they will be responsible with all of the other partners for the execution of all buy-outs. The funding of these buy-outs could also limit the cash available for distribution (in the future) to the remaining partners. The new physician does share equally in the increase in value of the entity from the date they buy-in.

If the group should decide to utilize this equity to debt conversion, then the partnership agreement for the group should also stipulate the priority of cash flows of the entity to protect departing members as well as providing distributions to senior physicians with greater equity before distributions to newer members with no notes payable. An example of the language which can be used in an Operating/Member Agreement is as follows:

- Under any buy-out structure, the medical real estate entity may want to consider a cap or maximum on the number of partners that can be bought out during the same calendar year. For example, if more than two partners are being bought out during any calendar year, the members shall proportionately share the buy-out value of only two partner buy-outs.

This provision is to protect the entity from having cash flow problems due to buy-outs of departing physicians. The departing physicians will still receive their full buy-out; however, the time frame will be extended. If the buy-out is to take place in the form of 10-year promissory notes, the "two buy-outs" limitation is applied to the value of two annual principal and interest note payments. If four physicians have left and are owed payments, they would share the value of two buy-outs among them and their 10-year notes could stretch out to any number of years beyond 10 years. The cap can be set at a percentage of annual gross revenue, net income, annual cash flow, or tied to a number of buy-outs as used in our example. Utilizing the cash flow cap is at the discretion of the entity if there is concern with respect to cash flow management. The medical real estate entity could also choose to execute a real estate bank refinance when the partner buy-out obligations due to the cap in place producing excessively long buy-out schedules for the departed partners.

One other item which will need to be documented, if the equity notes approach is utilized to facilitate the buy-in for new physicians is what happens on the sale of the building to an outside independent party, if the sale price is less than the amount needed to pay off the mortgage, equity notes, and equity. Sale proceeds would be distributed as follows:

1. Pay off bank debt and all other third-party debt
2. Pay equity of $75,000 per member
3. Pay off equity notes
4. Any proceeds remaining distributed equally among all members

Option 6: Use of Class A and Class B Units

Similar to the Equity Note Option described above, if the value grows to the point of not being affordable, and there is tremendous push back on coming up with the cash or even building entity financed loans, another option would be to consider the use of Class A and Class B units.

As with the equity note discussion in Option 5 above, when the founding members equity positions exceed some agreed upon value (i.e., $50,000 or some other agreed upon predetermined level), convert the existing equity greater than the targeted amount to Class B unit value for all current members so that each member is left with some of the equity.

This would leave the new buy-in amount at $50,000 per member for an equal Class A partnership interest. Another way of stating, all A units will have a value of $50,000 (which would be the cash buy-in for all new partners) and all equity above the $50,000 would be recorded as Class B unit value. This is similar to a refinance with the bank, but uses the existing partners as the bank with the establishment of the B units and their value. As you will see later in this section, there will be a payment for a return for the B unit values which recognize the built up equity over time.

1. The B units would pay a return equal to the same return on equity for all partners. For illustrative purposes, the rate of return is 6% (annual cash distributions as a percent of the real estate equity or value). Thus, both Classes of equity (A and B units) receive the 6% return. Since the Class B unit holders have more equity or value, they receive a greater portion of the annual distributions. This approach generally has each physician as an equal partner (or equal partner of the A units, which would be the voting units) but not equal equity or value and those with more equity receive a greater amount in terms of total annual distributions.
2. The A and B unit values are rolled into a note obligation that is only payable upon termination from the private practice orthopedic group practice entity and the corresponding termination from the real estate entity. Thus, it is not a demand note where a member can demand immediate payment.

The current partners will still get their value. The value is simply structured between A units and B unit value. The entity is still obligated to purchase the interest of departing members with that interest being purchased being the combination of the Class A unit value ($50,000) plus the Class B unit value on termination and the combination of the A and B unit values rolled into a note payable. While new members will pay less for an equal partnership interest, the issuance of the B units and the payment of B unit distributions will lessen the cash available for distribution, and thus the distributions are not equal per physician, but rather the same percent return on equity. While the new physician partners may pay less than the original partners to become a partner, they will receive less in annual cash distributions. However, from the day they become a Class A member, all growth in value from the day they become a partner will be equal among all Class A partners. This growth in value will be reflected in Class B units/value for the new partner and an increase in Class B units/value for the original partners or the partners. The Class B partners simply have a head start in their value and this gap is never closed under this approach.

By way of example, (assume six existing partners and one new partner) if on the next valuation date (after the new physician partner becomes partner (and thus now seven partners) and a new physician has presented themselves for partnership some number of years down the road (i.e., an eighth partner at the doorstep) and the value has increased by $350,000, the new partner (partner number seven) would now have Class B units equal to $50,000 in value and the original six partners would add $50,000 to each of their prior Class B values.

Another way to state this, all physicians receive an identical return on the $50,000 cash invested. In addition, they will be responsible with all of the other partners for the execution of all buy-outs. The funding of these buy-outs could also limit the cash available for distribution (in the future) to the remaining partners. One significant benefit to this Class A and Class B unit approach is the new physician (Class A unit holder) does share equally in the increase in value of the entity from the date they buy-in with all other Class A and Class B partners. The Class B unit holders have their difference in value recognized upon adoption of this approach, and all changes in value from this point forward are shared among all partners.

The other item which will need to be documented if the Class A and Class B units approach is utilized to facilitate the buy-in for new physicians and that is what happens on sale of the building to an outside independent party if the sale price is less than the amount needed to pay off the mortgage, Class B unit values and Class A unit values. Sale proceeds would be distributed

1. Pay off bank debt and all other third-party debt
2. Pay off Class A units/equity of $50,000 per member
3. Pay off Class B units/equity values
4. Any proceeds remaining distributed in proportion to class B unit values

In summary, medical practice real estate buy-ins present many challenges, but offer a potentially lucrative option with many available equity solutions.

References

1. Charles AG, Ortiz-Pujols S, Ricketts T, Fraher E, Neuwahl S, Cairns B, et al. The employed surgeon: a changing professional paradigm. JAMA Surg. 2013;148(4):323–8.
2. Bozic KJ, Roche M, Agnew SG. Hospital-based employment of orthopaedic surgeons--passing trend or new paradigm?: AOA critical issues. J Bone Joint Surg. 2012;94(9):e59.

Chapter 3
Setting up your Clinical Practice – Keys for Growth and Success

Eric C. Makhni and Brian Forsythe

Introduction

Believe it or not, most of your headaches as a new practitioner will not be related to clinical matters. They will be related to setting up, growing, maintaining, and troubleshooting your clinical practice. The key to building a successful clinical practice starts *before* you even accept your offer. Even as a seasoned surgeon, you will still be focusing on your practice development.

Part I: Before You Sign the Dotted Line

The foundation for your clinical practice begins far before you report to work on your first day. It actually begins much earlier, during your job search. The keys to finding the right practice for your individual goals and demands are covered elsewhere in this book, but hopefully you have located a practice that will help promote your growth and development, both from a clinical perspective and from a business perspective. Some things to consider when finalizing your practice include the following.

E. C. Makhni (✉)
Division of Sports Medicine, Department of Orthopedic Surgery, Henry Ford Health System, West Bloomfield, MI, USA

B. Forsythe
Rush University Medical Center, Department of Orthopedic Surgery, Chicago, IL, USA
e-mail: brian.forsythe@rushortho.com

E. C. Makhni et al. (eds.), *Orthopedic Practice Management*,
https://doi.org/10.1007/978-3-319-96938-1_3

Do They Actually Need Me Clinically?

The best way to get busy quickly (and therefore develop and mature clinically!) is to join a group that truly *needs* you from a clinical perspective. Therefore, it is best to ask your prospective partners if there is a clinical need for you, or will you be joining a crowded division that is unsure where you will fit in? (Helpful hint – if the partners in your division are actively recruiting you, as opposed to just the chairman or managing partner, it probably means they really need you to help with the clinical volume.)

Will You Be Set Up for Success, or Left on Your Own?

In order to build a successful clinical practice, you need to have assurances that your clinical team will grow as the volume grows. If the practice has a fair way of supporting team growth – mid-level providers, administrative assistance, hands in the OR – then you will be in good shape. On the contrary, if most of the partners are limited due to lack of team growth, then you will likely deal with the same issues.

Are You Restricted in What Types of Clinical Cases You Can See, or Are You Free to Practice Within the Scope of Your Subspecialty?

Ideally, your managing partners will tell you to feel free to build your clinical practice as you best see fit. But this may not always be the case. For example, in the sports medicine world, I was adamant in seeking out a practice that would not restrict the types of cases I would do. Many practices I encountered told me, "We would love to have you, but we really only want you operating on hips and knees." Or, "We would love to have you, but you can't do any of XX surgeries; those go to Dr. _____." In some instances, having a pre-determined focus may work perfectly for you if it matches your clinical interest or your burning desire to join a specific practice. However, for others, having such restrictions may limit your growth or, worse yet, your ability to build the type of practice you want.

Do Not Breeze Through the Negotiations Process!

Remember, you only get one chance to negotiate the terms of your contract. When you do get your offer sheet or initial contract, be sure to review it carefully and with the help of an attorney, as well as with the guidance of close colleagues or mentors.

You often only get one chance to submit your counter-terms, and if you don't recognize this, you may be stuck in a situation with sub-optimal terms and concessions, leaving considerable value on the table (and in the pocket of your practice!). And remember, if you want something, now is the time to ask! Once you start, there is little incentive for your managing partners to give you resources (that shiny new limb positioner or guaranteed block time). Therefore, get everything you can in writing before you start. You may not even have guaranteed office space unless get it in writing it ahead of time!

Part II: Before You Show Up for Work

There is a *lot* of time typically between the day you sign your contract and the day you actually see your first patient in the clinic. That means there is a *lot* of time for you to make sure you are prepared with what you need to ensure that you hit the ground running. There is nothing worse than having to delay your start date because of missed paperwork, delay in getting your license, and other nuances.

As soon as you sign your contract, it is imperative that you begin the licensing and credentialing process. It never ceases to amaze me how long this process actually takes. Not only do you have to jump through the hoops and red tape of your hospital credentialing process, but you also have to do the same at the state level in getting your medical license. For many, you may not be changing states from where you trained (or had your prior practice), and therefore you won't have to worry about the licensing process. However, for most of us, we do have to make sure we get new licensure. This process can take several months, and so you must begin the paperwork immediately. Often times there may be missing documentation that must be addressed, and each time the licensing body needs additional information, there is opportunity for lengthy delays.

Secondly, especially for new graduates, there is a deadline to get your hospital credentialing so that you can sit for your board exams at the earliest opportunity. Therefore, delays in hospital credentialing may disqualify you from timely board examination completion. Each hospital system has its own process from credentialing, and most require significant paperwork and reference letters. Therefore, no matter how busy you are, you must contact your hospital (and every hospital in your practice agreement) to begin the paperwork right away. And remember, there is a number of different items on the to-do list before you start that also needs to be scheduled and accounted for. Some health screens and EHR certifications/training require you to be on-site during certain days only. Therefore, you need to get all these dates well ahead of time so that you are able to not only schedule the dates you want but also so that you don't delay your target start date.

While the paperwork is being processed, the next task is to ensure that you are prepared to start your practice from the clinic and operating room perspective. If you are a current fellow or resident, now is the time to start collecting clinical protocols from your attendings. These include postoperative instructions, physical therapy protocols, and even how to perform special imaging sequences. If there are special x-ray views that you like, you need to make sure that your future clinic can get those views, and if they don't collect them already, it is helpful to connect the radiology manager with the manager from your training institution so that you can have continuity in your imaging protocols.

From a surgical perspective, there is a great deal to put together before you show up for your first day. First of all – do you have any guaranteed block time? This is the biggest obstacle for new surgeons as they begin their career. Lack of regularly scheduled block time (which is often the case for new surgeons) means that you will be adding cases on whenever you can. This can be disruptive to building a clinic schedule. Therefore, it is important to try to at least begin to have some regularity in the clinic with the hopes of similarly establishing it for the operating room. To make matters even more complicated, the clinic sites you are hired into may only have certain availability for your office hours. Therefore, you are likely going to be constrained in both aspects. Frequent conversation with your managing partners, nurse managers, and executive officers will no doubt help your transition and clinical forecasting.

In addition to securing actual operating *time*, you will need to secure your necessary operating *resources*. You may be entering a practice that has well-established resources with regards to implant type/contracts, assistants (first assists or residents), and beds/positioners. In this case, you may not have a lot of options. If you like to use a shoulder arthroplasty system by brand X, but your hospital is on contract with brands Y and Z, you will likely need to adapt your technique. However, if there are limb positioning devices, special bed attachments, or even individual tools or trays that you prefer or need to use, you must review this with the nurse manager of your product line well before you start. The hospital will be extremely reluctant to purchase new capital, even if you absolutely need it, and you need to be prepared for a lengthy approval process ahead. The hospital may try to avoid purchasing equipment outright, and instead insisting on renting that equipment for your cases. This may be acceptable, but consider the situation when you need to add a case on, or the equipment is not available for rent. Moreover, you need to make sure to think of *everything* you may need ahead of time. As with contract negotiations, the capital approval process is lengthy and resource-intense. The OR managers will not take kindly to submitting additional requests because you didn't realize there were additional equipment that you would need.

Another way to make sure your transition to the OR is seamless is to collect all the "pick lists" and case cards that you use in your fellowship or current practice and get them to your OR managers as soon as possible. This will allow them to review the lists to make sure all the small details can be accounted for when you arrive. One example from my own experience was that for tendon repairs (quad or patella tendon), I like to use large curved free needles to pass my suture with. Apparently, the hospital I joined did not have any of them, as the surgeons currently there used different passing methods. It took several weeks to get the needles in, and I had to improvise on several repairs until I got the equipment (however minor!) that I wanted. You will be surprised how difficult it is to get some of these basic instruments, so try to anticipate everything you will need well ahead of time.

Finally, the matter of block time must be settled. This is the most precious resource a new surgeon can secure. Often, your managing partner or chairman may "guarantee" you X number of days per week in the OR, but the hospital and OR managers may "guarantee" you something entirely different. In my situation, I was promised 1.5 days a week in the OR by my department, but the hospital was only willing to give me one half of one day a week (and that too, in the afternoon and following a surgeon who would be using morning block time). Thankfully, I had an extremely supportive department that was able to deliver on their promise. However, the process still took several weeks to sort through, and had I not brought the issue up months in advance, I would have been without block time for quite some time after starting.

For those of you who are not fortunate to get guaranteed block time from the beginning, or who are trying to secure additional block time, the best way to do so is to demonstrate need. Therefore, you must turn this obstacle upside down (for more on this valuable skill, please check out one of our favorite books of all time, and one suggested by Dr. Christopher Ahmad, entitled "The Obstacle is the Way", by Ryan Holiday) and use your free time in the clinic, seeing patients. The more patients you see, the more surgeries you will book, and the more the hospital will take notice. Be prepared to add cases on at the end of the day and on weekends, or better yet find a competing surgery center to send our business too. This will be the fastest way to gain more OR block time.

Part III: Getting Started – Patient Recruitment

The day finally arrives. You have your license. You have your hospital credentialing. You have your clinic schedule laid out, and you even have some block time. Now it's time to start seeing patients! But how will they find you?

Each practice has a different mechanism for directing patients to providers. As a fellow, the practice I trained at had a pool of surgeons in any given sub-specialty that was open to new patients, and the front office would simply rotate the incoming patient appointment requests through the pool of providers. In other systems, such as the one I joined, there was a large call center that tried to match up patient requests to surgeons based on clinical interests and preferences. Regardless of the system, the new surgeon must at least understand how patients make it to the clinic. These referrals are relatively *passive*, meaning that the patients will come onto the schedule without any active effort on your part (besides letting the call center know that you are alive and accepting patients). In some cases, this may be enough to grow your practice, especially if you are the only provider in a given sub-specialty or are coming to a practice that has a large need for a certain type of provider (e.g. someone who takes care of shoulder patients). However, for many of us, this is not the case, and while the passive method for practice growth may help, it will not allow us to expeditiously build a practice of our desire.

The most efficient way to build a practice is to do so actively. This approach embodies the entrepreneurial spirit. The particular approach depends largely on your sub-specialty, but for most elective disciplines (joint replacement, sports medicine, spine, hand, foot/ankle), the approach is relatively similar. First and foremost, you must prescribe to the "Three A's" of Availability, Affability, and Ability. In order to build a successful practice, you *must* be Available. This means keeping your schedule flexible to add patients and making it easy for patients to get on your schedule. Open up weekend and evening clinics. You should see any patient that comes to the door, no matter what the chief complaint is. You should never turn down a patient from a potential referral source, even if you know that patient will not really need your services (but at least you can help guide the patient to someone that will be more appropriate). In our field of sports medicine, that means giving your cell phone number out to physical therapists, athletic trainers, and school officials so that there is *always* a quick and easy way to get patients in for evaluations. I remember a colleague of mine who was new in practice and who actually turned patients away from a primary care provider because he didn't think the patient required surgery (he instead referred the patient away to a nonoperative provider without even seeing the patient). Not only did that colleague lose the opportunity to meet a new patient, but he also turned off the referring provider who confided to me that they would never refer patients to my colleague again. Once you are available and starting to meet patients, then you also absolutely must fulfill the second and third of the A's (affability and ability), but those won't ever matter if you can't get patients through the door! Being affable entails being personable and agreeable to patients. Simple pears in achieving this include listening to patients as they explain their health problems, sitting at eye level with your patients, and other basics of good physician–patient communication. And finally, being able means that you still have to do a good job with your clinical care! Good indications and outcomes will help your practice grow organically and lead to a waiting room of happy (or at least reasonably so) patients.

Another strategy to actively grow your practice is through outreach and networking. Each hospital often has "meet and greets" for new providers who enter the system. In fact, the hospital actually facilitates these *just* so that the specialists can meet the primary care providers! Obviously, getting to know your colleagues in primary care will help in meeting new providers who may want to refer to you, but remember – primary care providers also want to meet specialists whom they trust so that they can ensure their patients receive top-notch care! You should actively try to meet providers with whom you work so that you can additionally establish seamless and efficient lines of communication. This will enable enhanced patient care, because you very much need their help as well!

Finally, no matter how long you have been in practice, you must always try to provide good communication to those who refer patients to you. I recommend always sending a copy of your office note to the provider who referred to the patient to you. This allows the provider to be up to date with what is going on with his/her patient, which will in turn give extra confidence to the patient of the care team. Don't forget to shoot a quick note, email, or other type of message to your peers so that they know you have established care for their patients.

Additionally, one of the best ways to get your name out there is to literally get your name out there. This means being very active with giving lectures. As a sports medicine doctor, I spent countless hours giving talks at department meetings, resident lectures, physical therapy clinics, primary care (adult and pediatrics grand rounds), emergency department grand rounds – anywhere and any time I could! I also went out on trips with the hospital outreach team to meet local primary care providers to introduce myself as well. You would be surprised how hard it can be to actually get your name out there, and; that even doing all this still may require continued work throughout the first several years of your practice.

Finally, no matter how much outreach you do, how many lectures you give, and how many sporting events you cover, the best way to build your practice is organically. Take good care of your patients. Communicate well with them. Treat them as if they were your own family. *Always* act in their best interest. Eventually, this behavior will be rewarded not only with happy patients and good outcomes but also with referrals from your most valuable referral sources: your patients!

Part IV: Your Online Presence

Whether you like it or not, we live in a very connected world. Your patients – and anyone else for that matter – can find out your educational background, CV, and anything else about you through the web. That means that many of your prospective patients will be looking you up before they meet you and even after they meet you but before they confirm their trip to the operating room. The information out there on the web is accessible to all and *will* be investigated, especially if you are new in practice without an established patient base. Understanding how the online world works for physicians will help when it comes time to influence what is out there about you.

There are many avenues by which your online presence is broadcast. Your practice or department will no doubt include you in their webpage, and so please make sure your information is all current and up to date. There are also numerous third party organizations that broadcast your licensing and academic backgrounds. Be careful – some of these pull information from your licensing and credentialing applications and may actually include your home phone number and address!

One easy way to directly influence the information online about you is by having your own professional web page. You should of course consult your program or department regarding rules about individual pages, especially if not through your health care system. However, having your own page is a very effective way of marketing and clinical care in that you can provide targeted information about your practice – procedures you do, office and surgery locations, insurances accepted, and so forth – as well as your clinical protocols (postoperative instructions, physical therapy protocols, and patient guides). Additionally, you can highlight your research efforts, patient education guides, and even blog posts that all contribute to helping your web page gain visibility in search engines (a.k.a. "SEO," or Search Engine Optimization) that ultimately helps guide patients to your website (and to you!). Augments to your web page can include social media accounts, and this is discussed extensively in a separate chapter. Of course, be careful to pay heed to hospital policy as well as patient privacy laws when posting information on these sites.

With most of these options, the provider has numerous opportunities to influence his/her online presence. However, there are some media that are entirely out of the control of orthopedic providers. These include online patient reviews. For better or worse, physicians are treated just like consumer stores and products, in that they are reviewed online and given anywhere from one to five stars for their perceived level of service. There is significant controversy regarding this rating system, especially if used as an actual metric of physician quality. You can easily imagine a hard-working, caring physician who scores low on a patient feedback score because of a rude front-office staff, or an unethical and incompetent physician scoring five stars because of a cheerful patient interaction in the office. Nevertheless, these ratings systems exist, and in large numbers. Popular sites include Healthgrades, Vitals, and even Yelp and Google. Try as you might, you may not make everyone happy, and therefore you are vulnerable to unhappy patient reviews. The main way to counter this is to try to promote a high-quality experience for the patient, beginning with their first contact with the office (your secretary, your scheduler, or even the call center which you unfortunately have little control over), and carrying into their experience with you (and your team!) in the office and before/after surgery. As with the consumer world, you only need one unfavorable outcome or interaction to bring down your average quality ratings online, and so it is perfectly reasonable to provide information to all of your patients on how they can leave feedback for you online so that you can hope to have a representative sampling online of patient feedback. In our practice, and in many others that I am aware of, all patients are provided with cards that provide not only contact information or other helpful information regarding the practice but also different ways to leave feedback online for the physician.

Part V: Never Forget the Basics!

Hopefully, following the above advice will help you take your first steps toward efficiently and effectively growing your practice. Never forget, however, that your practice is built upon the backs of not only you, but your entire team. It is critical that you work hard to respect your team members of all levels, because unhappy team members will yield inferior results in patient care and satisfaction. Just like you work hard for your bosses that are kind and caring to you, so will your team if you are kind and caring to them. Promote a healthy office environment, and one in which your team – no matter what level they are – can offer feedback to you as well. Failure to do so will promote a propagation of errors and inefficiencies that will only hurt you and the practice down the road. There is a wealth of information out there in the forms of books, podcasts, and journals, which will help you learn to be a good team leader. Unfortunately, this critical skill is not taught in any scope in medical school or residency, and so you have to learn it either through your own scholarship or through trial and error. I recommend more of the former.

Recommended Reading

1. Ahmad CS. SKILL: 40 principles that surgeons, athletes, and other elite performers use to achieve mastery. Paperback – 1 June 2015.
3. Carnegie D, MacMillan A. How to win friends & influence people. 17 Sep 2004; Unabridged.
2. Holiday R. The obstacle is the way: the timeless art of turning trials into triumph. 2014.

Chapter 4
Recruiting and Incorporating Mid-Level Providers

Peter Borowsky, Jacob Blanchett, Kyle Pilz, and Eric C. Makhni

Synergy: [Sin-er-jee]: noun: The interaction of the elements that, when combined, produce a total effect that is greater than the sum of the individual elements, contributions.

Timeline and Trends in Physician Extender Usage

For more than 50 years, mid-level practitioners (MLPs) have been augmenting medical practice in an effort to improve and expand healthcare reach. It was in the mid-1960s that physicians and educators recognized the relative shortage of primary care physicians. In an effort to address this deficit, Eugene Stead, MD of Duke University Medical Center established the first class of physician assistants in 1965. Four Navy Hospital corpsmen (heavily trained in various medical practices from their extensive military services) comprised that inaugural class in 1967. Similarly, it was in 1965 that Dr. Loretta Ford and Dr. Henry Silver developed the first nurse practitioner (NP) program at the University of Colorado.

Today, approximately 115,500 certified physician assistants (PAs) and 222,000 nurse practitioners (NPs) practice in medical and surgical subspecialties in all 50 states, the District of Columbia, US territories, and the uniform services [1, 2]. Both nurse practitioners and physician assistants hold prescription privileges, including controlled substances in all 50 states and the District of Columbia [1, 3]. Both physician assistants and nurse practitioners are in heavy demand as they represent a formidable option in the ongoing mission to provide affordable and accessible health care to millions of aging Americans. Three-quarters of physician assistants receive multiple job offers upon passing their initial licensing and certification

P. Borowsky · J. Blanchett · E. C. Makhni (✉)
Division of Sports Medicine, Department of Orthopedic Surgery, Henry Ford Health System, West Bloomfield, MI, USA
e-mail: pborows1@hfhs.org; jblanch3@hfhs.org

K. Pilz
RUSH University Medical Center, Department of Sports Medicine, Midwest Orthopedics at RUSH, Chicago, IL, USA
e-mail: kyle.pilz@rushortho.com

E. C. Makhni et al. (eds.), *Orthopedic Practice Management*,
https://doi.org/10.1007/978-3-319-96938-1_4

exams [1]. Named in 2015 as one of the "most promising jobs in America" by *Forbes* and *US Today*, the PA profession has seen its demand for PAs increase by greater than 300% between 2011 and 2014 [4]. Nurse practitioners have watched their field experience similar growth with an estimated 22,000 NPs completing their programs in 2014–2015 [5].

Why Incorporate an MLP?

Benefits of MLP Utilization

Nurse practitioners, physician assistants, and athletic trainers benefit medical practice in various ways. Applying the help of mid-level practitioners effectively can produce benefits for both the patient and the practice.

Patient-Related Benefits

Studies have shown that when MLPs are part of the healthcare team, hospital readmission rates and length of stay decrease [6]. A Harris poll survey demonstrated 93% satisfaction rates among Americans who interact with PAs. In this poll, 92% responded that having a PA makes it easier to obtain an appointment and 91% believe that PAs improve the quality of health care [7]. In a patient satisfaction survey conducted in 2011, nurse practitioners outscored physicians [3]. In 15 of the 18 core questions asked in the survey, there was a statistically significant difference in favor of nurse practitioners [3, 8]. A Kaiser Permanente Center for Health Research study on physician assistants illustrated an 89–96% overall patient satisfaction with PAs. The satisfaction scores were in regards to level of interpersonal care, patient confidence in provider, and provider understanding of patient problems [9].

Productivity-Related

A socioeconomic monitoring system survey by the AMA found that physicians who employed nonphysician practitioners were able to work 1 week less per year, on average [10]. These physicians observed an increased number of hours available for office visits and an average of 18% increased net income [10]. These physicians found greater practice efficiency, ability to extend their practice, and re-distribution of their scope of practice to more desirable areas [10].

With a PA or NP on staff, practices see reduced patient waiting times, increased clinical throughput, and increased patient access to care through increase in number of office locations, increased hours, and improved accessibility/patient correspondence [1]. These practices also reported improved patient compliance and continuity of care [1, 3].

Special Considerations Before Incorporating the MLP: Cost of Hiring and "Maintaining" a Mid-Level Practitioner – Salary, Benefits, Continued Education, Licensure, and Insurance Considerations

The incorporation of a mid-level practitioner to their practice is not something every physician will find amenable to their personality and individual needs. There are several considerations that must be addressed before incorporating MLPs to any given practice.

Costs of Hiring and "Maintaining" MLPs

When considering the total financial cost entailed with adding the MLP to the practice, there are several inclusions that must be taken into account. In addition to the base salary the physician extender will earn, an additional 25–35% will be added in benefits, continuing medical education (CME) provisions, licensure, and malpractice insurance. According to the Medical Group Management Association (MGMA), physician assistants generate revenues greater than what their compensation costs the employer. Most recent reports demonstrate that for every dollar of charges the PA generates for the practice, the employer pays on average 30 cents to employ the PA [11].

Benefit packages including the health insurance, dental, vision, life insurance, short- and long-term disability options, etc. will cost the employer an average of $1000–2000 per mid-level practitioner annually. Liability insurance policies paid by provider can range from $1500 to $2000 paid annually. Typically, the employer will cover the cost associated with state licensure, DEA licenses through the professional regulatory body, and national and specialty board annual dues. The sum total of these "start-up" costs to the practice of each mid-level provider, therefore, can range from $3000 to $5000.

The majority of PAs will carry malpractice insurance under their supervising physician's policy. There is an option to carry one's own malpractice insurance, a trend seeing growing popularity. Nurse practitioners will carry their own malpractice insurance due to the absence of a delegated supervising physician [3].

There will be other expenses involved in the recruitment and hiring of a PA, NP, or ATC, and these primarily entail the interview process and the myriad aforementioned start-up expenses. The cost involved with the recruitment phase of an MLP will typically be limited to reimbursement of travel expenses and lodging associated with the interview process only. Signing bonuses for mid-level practitioners are rare. Going forward, the combination of regular salary and benefits paid on behalf of the practitioner typically totals 1.25–1.375x the annual base salary.

Liability Issues

These include responsibilities, malpractice, supervision, and delegation of prescriptive authority.

Before incorporating MLPs into the practice, several other considerations remain on the part of the hiring physician or group. These include issues pertaining to terminal responsibility, the increased financial burden of malpractice insurance, and the ever-present issue with practice supervision involving the mid-level practitioner. In addition, the delegation of prescriptive authority is another issue that needs to be discussed with the group and the MLP themselves. PAs will maintain their own DEA number; however, it is at the discretion of the physician and the MLP to construct the specific prescriptive spectrum within which the PA or NP will work. Some practices and/or physicians will elect to limit the delegation of prescriptive authority for schedule II narcotics, for instance, or possibly all controlled substances.

Recruiting a Mid-Level Practitioner

Recruitment Avenues

Direct Referral

In many instances, the most comfortable means of "first contact" with a prospective mid-level petitioner is the direct referral by another trusted known party within the practice. Oftentimes, employers and hiring physicians find great comfort in developing a recent graduate who performed student clerkship within the practice, grew up in the community of one of the partner physicians or other clinicians, or maintained some other level of relationship prior to entering their graduate medical program.

Farm System

Similar to a major league baseball team developing its "in-house" talent at the minor league level with hopes of one day reaping the benefits of that training as it manifests at the major league level, a medical practice also recruits mid-level practitioners in similar ways. Similar to the "direct referral" concept, physician assistants, athletic trainers, and nurse practitioners often "rise through the ranks" from a prior position within the practice. These clinicians often served in prior roles as research assistants, medical assistants, or other miscellaneous physician extender roles. Again, this means of introduction allows for the comfort of a known entity and an individual that has been vetted based on prior experience, observation of behavior, and work ethic, etc.

Third-Party Recruiter

The nurse practitioner looking for a job opportunity has myriad options today. Sites such as AdvancedPractice.com, Monster.com, NPJobs.com, Indeed.com, and StaffCare.com (to name a few) offer both full-time and locum tenens (temporary) and contract-to-hire job opportunities. Similarly, PAs utilizing sites such as PAJobSite.com, HealtheCareers.com, BartonAssociates.com, CareerBuilder.com, and AAPA.org also will find a similar array of opportunities. These sites provide a starting point for both candidate and employer and can also comprehensively help govern the entire job search and employment process. Similarly, third-party "head-hunters" provide yet another avenue for access to PA and NP job opportunities both regionally and nationally. The use of a third-party recruitment service for this purpose will cost a medical practice an average of $200 per job posting. Human resources departments at a medical practice utilize and compile information and resumes through all of the above sources in an effort to find the most qualified and appropriate candidates to meet a practice's needs. When initiating the hunt, the HR director is the most sensible starting point to kick-start a candidate search to fill any mid-level provider position.

Retained Student Trainee

Simply stated, occasionally one finds a gem right under their nose and can be fortunate enough to higher the PA, nurse practitioner, or other graduate student training directly with them or with a partner. There is certainly no easier way to have a candidate vetted than to have witnessed their work directly during student clerkship or to have had one of your colleagues do that for you. This avenue undoubtedly provides the comfort of knowing the prospective hire has already seen the practice "from the inside" and has an accurate and full understanding of what environment, workload hours, and practice dynamics they are getting themselves into.

Recruitment Considerations

Timelines/Urgency of Need

A major factor in the decision of hiring a PA, nurse practitioner, or athletic trainer is certainly the level of urgency in filling the position. Often times, a prior clinician has left unexpectedly, thus leaving behind an increased workload for others. Even when a clinician's departure is well planned and anticipated, it often is only forewarned by 4–12 weeks in most occasions, thus creating a semi-urgent initiation of candidate searches, job postings, and word of mouth search for the best available PA, NP, or other candidates. The timeline and urgency of need to fill the position certainly can create limitations in the candidate pool size and possibly risk a physician being in the position where they feel obligated to make a hire during a time of year when the recent graduate pool may be more limited. For example, a large majority of physician assistant programs have graduation dates in the spring and summer months, and candidates typically complete board certification in the 1 month after graduation and are available for hire and to begin employment 6–8 weeks after graduation at the earliest.

Practice Needs

A major factor in the PA and NP hiring process is the specific need the practice is trying to fulfill. In many instances, a physician or group of physicians has decided that they would like a qualified clinician who is able to diagnose and treat, but will be serving in a direct "extender" role in clinic. This would imply the PA or NP is physically with the physician in office, clinic, and/or OR, indirectly augmenting the daily management of the practice in this regard. In this role, athletic trainers will commonly function in the "physician extender" capacity, augmenting clinic days with evaluation and management of patients, as well as applying their clinical experience with management of patient phone calls, emails, and provision of patient education in clinic including physical therapy prescriptions, patient Q&A, gait training with crutches, brace application, and other miscellaneous tasks directly under the supervision of the physician on premises. In contrast, the hiring physician may know their need mandates the hiring of a more autonomous clinical practitioner that will see patients independently. This may range from a fully independent clinic at a satellite location run without supervision to a single day of clinic with the physician present on an intermittent basis. When the need for an autonomous practitioner is paramount, the nurse practitioner can fulfill this role to the maximal level of autonomy, meaning the NP can practice independently under their own license, manage, treat, diagnose, and carry out clinical practice without the need for a legally appointed supervising position. The PA can perform their clinical responsibilities independently at a similar level, but there needs to be a delegated supervising physician on record and available to with whom to correspond on an as-needed basis. The personal needs and availability of the hiring physician regarding their anticipated level of on-site versus remote supervision will dictate a lot in the decision in whom and how to incorporate when it comes time to search for a mid-level practitioner.

Willingness to Delegate

Hiring and utilizing a nurse practitioner, physician assistant, or athletic trainer is certainly not something that will apply, nor even be appropriate, for all physicians or practices. For instance, a physician who only wants to simply obtain help with patient volume and administrative minutia may benefit most from help provided by a medical assistant, more office administrative help, or refining their utilization of their EHR system or dictation. Simply stated, some physicians or medical groups simply prefer not to delegate clinical decision-making, prescriptive authority, surgical and clinical responsibility, etc., and never will. For these individuals, it simply may not be necessary to employee an NP, PA, nor ATC simply because it is incongruent with their goals, values, or unnecessary given their personal practice needs.

For the remainder of physicians who do wish to delegate some of their clinical responsibility and decision-making in order to offload any myriad aspects of their practice, there are several considerations. These doctors will need to scrutinize their level of willingness and comfort to delegate prescriptive authority, certain aspects of surgery, and what level and volume of their patient population they wish the mid-level practitioner to see independently. The most common "low-hanging fruit" physicians will elect to delegate include global period visits, noncomplex joint injections, and pre-op visits. This, in aggregate, displaces a substantial volume in most practices and thus allows for the physician to take on an increased number of new patient visits and/or spend more time on complex cases, a welcome shift in time appropriation.

Applicant Selection

The importance of the recruitment, evaluation, and screening process cannot be overstated. As with any hire in the business world, it is difficult to make a well-informed decision on an individual with such a limited amount of contact in most cases. As a result, it is certainly of utmost importance to have a system for screening, contacting, and communicating with the potential applicants and active candidates during the applicant selection process. Equally as important is the vetting of any references and exploration of any and all available personal and work history.

Screening of Applicants

Depending on ongoing workload and personal desires, some physicians or practices will prefer to screen their own applicants' curriculum vitae, while some will simply rely on the initial screen to be done by their human resources department. The initial decision needs to be made whether one wants all potential applicant resumes to come for screening to their inbox or to be weeded out by HR staff or other practice representative. Unless the applicant is a well-vetted graduate or former student/employee with whom there is a preexisting relationship and arrives at your practice's "front doorstep" ready to work, the initial phase of screening is essentially blind, and the level of information and comfort garnered from the initial review of resumes is only as good as the quality of information therein.

Initial Contact

Once the initial applicants' CVs have been reviewed, the "initial contact" can be in the form of a mailed letter, email, or phone call. Again, this initial contact can be made by anyone from the HR director, an HR representative, or someone from the practice including the hiring physician, another physician extender, or even an administrative assistant involved in the hiring process. Certainly, this initial contact is of utmost important, as it represents the first impression of the practice upon the applicant. Naturally, there is an exchange of introductions and discussion regarding salient points of the practice and the candidate's CV, but there really is one paramount purpose to the initial contact: Do you want to meet this applicant in person or not?

First Exposure: Impressions

Once the decision is made to pursue a given applicant further and meet in person, there are various ways to take the next step in the process. Many physicians prefer a formal face-to-face sit-down "interview" in an office setting. This traditional format certainly allows for conversation in a private setting without distractions. It also allows for more informal expounding and follow-up of initial topics highlighted in the initial phone or email contact. A face-to-face sit-down interview allows for at least some level of assessment of an applicant's comfort with an unfamiliar environment, mannerisms, eye contact, and other personal tendencies, positive or negative. At some point, however, the benefits of the face-to-face sit-down interview plateau and the physician/clinician interviewer must decide if there will be added value in the applicant observing the practice in action firsthand.

Alternatively, personal preference or a busy practice schedule may not allow for the time needed for a face-to-face interview. The only option may be to have the candidate's first contact with the practice in an observation role during an active workday. Some physicians prefer to follow a face-to-face interview with a "second interview" entailing direct observation, whereas some physicians might decide to forego the face-to-face interview and have the candidate observe clinic or surgical cases directly in order to experience a sampling of the "real life" practice in person and carry out the interview in the form of further discussion "on the fly." In many fields, but especially in medicine, there is a significant value in allowing applicants to see the practice running on all cylinders, whether it be in the midst of a busy clinic day, managing surgical cases in the operating room, making phone calls, responding to emails, or any combination thereof. This certainly requires the hiring physician to be "comfortable in their own skin" enough to allow an applicant to see all aspects of the practice from the inside. Without this opportunity, however, one can only guess what a candidate's level of understanding will be in regards to the scope of practice and everyday rigors of the position they seek.

First Impressions: Exposure and Disclosure

It is only natural for a provider to want to put on a nice presentation for a potential hire. At the same time, however, it is equally ideal to give any candidate an accurate idea of "reality" and allow for some level of sampling of real life in the practice. The amount of information disclosed to an applicant and the level of exposure that one will allow during the interview process obviously need to be made based on the hiring physician's comfort level and personality. Unfortunately, in most cases the timeline of both parties will typically not allow for a 2- to 4-week period of intense observation and personal interaction in a physically challenging and sleep deprived state; however, it is the personal opinion of this chapter's author that the closer the hiring practice can come to this during the process, the better.

Vetting/Referral Verification

Without the ability to spend a substantial amount of time together to "feel things out" before deciding on a potential hire, there is increased reliance on the applicant's references and those individuals or groups with the most prior contact and interaction with the candidate. Discussion with the least-biased individuals with whom the applicant spent time can produce a better understanding of the person's strengths, weaknesses, and tendencies. Even if the only available references for an applicant are those produced by the candidate themselves, a conversation with these individuals can often elucidate helpful information about the prospect's work ethic, attitude, punctuality, and other personal traits.

Naturally, a practice or employer can only garner so much information on a potential hire before making a commitment one way or the other. Much like with any relationship, the legitimacy of the first impressions will either be belied or validated once a more substantial amount of quality time is spent together.

The Hiring Process

Offer

The manner in which the actual extension of a job offer takes place for a mid-level practitioner is highly variable, but the primary purpose of the message is typically the same: join our team and please come ASAP. By the time a formal offer is made, the majority, if not all, of the details have been sorted out. Typically, a discussion has been had with both the prospective employer and the HR department regarding salary, benefits, bonus structure, continuing education allowance, paid time off, and all other related details. The timing of the actual start date is highly variable as well, ranging from the next day to several months down the road. An NP or PA who is already credentialed, licensed, and with DEA number might literally be available for work the day following the hire and begin processing paperwork and initiate the privileges and credentialing process. On the other hand, a newly graduated practitioner may still have yet to complete their respective national board exam, wait for results, and then submit official paperwork for state licensure, hospital privileges, etc. This often may create a waiting period of 90–180 days for the new clinician to be fully credentialed and able to deliver direct patient care and bill for services.

Contract

The use of a formal employment contract is a common, but not required, practice for mid-level practitioners and their employers. Approximately, 60% of physician assistants practicing in orthopedic surgery have active employment contracts [12]. Written contracts, while commonly viewed negatively by the employee as binding and restrictive, actually are valuable for providing protection for both the clinician and the employer. The practice new to hiring mid-level clinicians will benefit from the services of an attorney with experience in PA and NP contracts. Similarly, it would behoove the prospective clinician greatly to retain legal consult for purposes of contract review and guidance with any negotiation. Most commonly, a candidate physician assistant or nurse practitioner will manage their own negotiation with the practice's human resources department, but certainly having an attorney well versed in these contracts available for consult can only help.

Employment contracts for mid-level practitioners may or may not include length of contract terms. The common fear among MLPs regarding contract terms is that the contract is binding for 24–36 months at a time and contract material cannot be addressed during the term of the contract. This is an important point that needs to be confirmed by both parties prior to final agreements. There are myriad resources for athletic trainers, nurse practitioners, and physician assistants seeking employment and/or contract negotiation advice on the respective professional websites. AANP.org, AAPA.org, and NATA.org provide excellent "career center" resources for both employer and employee to gain insight into the job search and hiring process. On these sites, one can find specifics and guidelines regarding pertinent contract inclusions such as benefits, continuing education allotment, paid time off structure, malpractice insurance, profit sharing, profession dues, disability insurance, non-compete covenants, and termination clauses.

Board Certification

Upon graduation, nearly every new graduate nurse practitioner and physician assistant will have their national board certification exam scheduled soon thereafter, knowing they must leap that one last proverbial final hurdle before joining the "real world" and beginning their new career. Similarly, this sometimes awkward waiting period will leave a hiring physician or practice waiting for the exam results in order to "onboard" their new clinician and finalize submission of credentialing paperwork and requested privileges.

Prospective employers can be encouraged by relatively healthy pass rates for NPs, ATCs, and PAs national board exams for the first time. In the most recent four certification years 2012–2016 of the NATA BOC exam (National Athletic Trainers' Association Board of Certification), athletic trainers have maintained a pass rate ranging between 80 and 82% [13]. Over the same time frame, first-time physician assistant and nurse practitioners have passed their respective board certification exams at a 93–96% and 75–89% rate, respectively [14].

Training and Integrating a New Mid-Level Practitioner

Learning Curve - Setting Expectations and Goals

It is the obligation of the supervising physician to decide what level of autonomy he/she wishes to allow the MLP to maintain in practice. The general outline of expectations for how the clinician will be utilized on a daily basis should be highlighted as early as possible in the interview process. Some physicians seek only an "extender" to serve as a scribe in clinic, assist with evaluation of patients to improve clinic throughput, and manage patient correspondence responding to phone calls and email. Conversely, some physicians expect their nurse practitioner or physician assistant to maintain their own patient volume, manage an independent volume in clinic, and oversee their own billing and collections. In the 2016 practice survey of the Physician Assistants in Orthopedic Surgery (PAOS), only 28.4% of respondents reported having access to their own billing and collections data. 56% of the PAs responding see patients exclusively on their own, with another 33% seeing patients both on their own and with their supervising physician at some point. In effect, only 11% of PAs are seeing patients exclusively in conjunction with the physician [12]. Clearly, the trend of physician assistant usage in the orthopedic practice is to extend clinical availability and reach, as opposed to simply augmenting the physician's practice together in the same place and time. Regardless of what base structure of MLP utilization the physician desires to uphold, these expectations and goals should be addressed early and often, putting goals and thresholds in writing and kept someplace where they can be readily reviewed.

Active Versus Passive Training - See One, Do One, Teach One

As with the development of any skill set, the on-the-job training of a practicing orthopedic ATC, NP, or PA can happen in many different ways. Tasks with less associated potential liability, such as dictation of patient notes and patient correspondence such as phone calls or emails, might be delegated immediately upon hire. Clinic notes can be reviewed and amended before becoming an official part of the patient's chart. Other clinical skills such as joint injection or cast application will likely be learned first through observation of the supervising physician or other experienced clinician, and then modeled for the mentor and "taught back" on several occasions before the skill is then applied autonomously. This "see one, do one, teach one" allows for more complete confidence in the clinician's skill set on the part of both practitioners. In addition, Joint Commission accredited hospitals are required to include PAs and NPs in their standardized focused professional practice evaluations (FPPE) and ongoing professional practice evaluations (OPPE) administered by the medical staff office annually or semi-annually. Intended to ensure continued clinical competence among providers, the documentation of these skill sets will be required for the provider to maintain them among their approved privileges in the medical center.

As a hiring physician, one should be aware of their respective hospital's requirements for the attestation of the MLPs competence in their respective set of desired "core" and "specialty" privileges. Some medical centers will allow for the vetting of the provider's competency in clinical skills to be conducted by a peer PA or NP, whereas other centers require the documentation to be rendered by the supervising physician. Alternatively, hospitals may also utilize systems that track provider clinical activity or collect specific date through programs such as the Physician Quality Reporting System (PQRS) or the Surgical Care Improvement Project (SCIP) [1]. Additionally, medical practices might obligate a given fraction of continuing education credits be specific to the provider's subspecialty.

Aside from direct one-on-one training with the supervising physician, several other options exist for new or experienced clinicians to both develop new skill sets and refine current techniques, both in the clinical and surgical setting.

When to "Lengthen the Leash"

Each physician or surgeon is unique in their appetite to allow others to render care on their behalf. The level of autonomy bestowed upon a physician assistant in orthopedic surgery ranges from independent surgery with remote supervision to as minimal as simply assisting with seeing patients in clinic [1, 15, 16]. Similarly, the scope of practice of nurse practitioners may consist of a solo practice without physician supervision, delivering patient care directly alongside a managing physician, or any combination thereof [17]. Just as with training orthopedic residents, the decision to allow the nurse practitioner or physician assistant more clinical or surgical autonomy is made when certain skill set thresholds are met and demonstrated to the physician consistently with competency. Every effort should be made by the hiring physician to clearly communicate just how far their comfort level spans with allowing the physician extender to broaden their scope of autonomous practice as they progress in training. Granted, not every mid-level practitioner needs to do surgery independently to be satisfied professionally, but it is the personal experience of this author that even a little goes a long way.

Maximizing Utilization of Mid-Level Practitioners

Goals - Bigger Versus Better

Maybe the principal question that needs to be answered when an orthopedic practice decides to incorporate a mid-level provider is whether the primary objective is to increase patient volume or improve practice efficiency. Physicians employing PAs or NPs report more flexible, forgiving work schedules [11]. They also find greater practice efficiency, improved access to care for patients, and an expanded practice [10]. With a mid-level practitioner on staff, there exists an immediate new potential to see more patients in the same amount of time, or see the same number of patients in even less time than before.

Expanded Reach

With the addition of a nurse practitioner or physician assistant to the practice, the physician also may elect to extend clinic hours or expand their services to additional clinic sites. The resulting greater access to care for patients via the broadened practice provides better ease of scheduling and increased patient volume [10]. An orthopedic practice planning expansion in this manner should anticipate the increased volume of not only surgical cases but the resultant surge in clinic follow-up visits and associated hike in patient correspondence and related administrative burden. Certainly, there is a ripple effect of both increased volume and expanded reach to be accounted for before the business benefits can be realized.

Efficiency Considerations

As found in the AMA Socioeconomic Monitoring System Survey of 2012, physicians who employed nonphysician practitioners were able to work 1 week less per year on average. With a PA, NP, or ATC on staff, practices enjoy improved efficiency marked by reduced patient wait times and increased clinic throughput [1, 3, 18]. Assuming there is only a single PA or NP working with the orthopedic surgeon, a personnel decision must be made regarding whether to utilize the clinician in the operating room or in clinic seeing additional patients. Here, the physician must truly demonstrate their prioritization on either surgical efficiency versus increased clinic availability. A case can certainly be made to support either model. If the NP or PA is able to see initial post-op visits, simple joint injection patients, and assess new patients with recent injuries, this creates more available clinic time for the physician to accommodate more complex cases or conduct other business, etc.

In some scenarios, physician preference may be to simply reduce overall workload and administrative burden. Here, the use of a trained physician extender may be the missing piece of the puzzle, as NPs, ATCs, and PAs all are capable of responsibly and efficiently managing patient emails, phone calls, patient paperwork, and reviewing patient records. Many physicians cite the intangible benefit of simply having a clinician available in the office for patient-related concerns and other clinically oriented issues beyond the scope of the administrative staff.

Patient Considerations

There are several notable and well-documented patient-related benefits to having an MLP on staff with the orthopedic practice, as highlighted at the beginning of this chapter. None of these benefits can be realized, however, without the physician's empowerment of that practitioner to their patients on a regular basis. Despite improving trends in patient acceptance to see PAs and NPs as primary providers, studies have still shown patient preference in favor of seeing resident physicians over nonphysician providers [19]. Because of these inherent tendencies among patients, a supervising physician must make it a daily habit to reinforce to new patients the MLPs expertise, credibility, and their important role as a partner in delivering care in that practice. In many instances, the physician extender may be conducting the initial office visit, and therefore the opportunity for appropriate introductions and professional endorsement of the clinician on the part of the physician may not exist. As a result, any physician employing ATCs, NPs, or PAs on staff should consider including a video, intro letter, or other medium on their practice website or equivalent welcome paperwork for purposes of explaining the role of the MLP in their practice.

Revenue

While the decision to hire a mid-level practitioner may or may not be financially motivated, there are myriad avenues through which to generate substantial revenue directly through the services of an ATC, NP, or PA in the orthopedic practice. According to Medical Group Management Association, physician assistant charges, on average, triple the same PAs cost to employer [20]. Based on 2016 data, the average primary care nurse practitioner total annual income of $108,000 was dwarfed by their average annual collections of over $347,000 [21]. The effectiveness of nurse practitioners is augmented when they are assisted by ancillary staff. A 2014 study demonstrated significant improvements in both productivity and cost-effectiveness of NPs practicing in the primary care setting when provided with medical assistant (MA) support [22]. Furthermore, when comparing the utilization of medical assistants to athletic trainers in the physician extender role, a 2013 study published in Sports Health showed statistically significant improvements in both patient encounters (18–22%) and total collections (10–60%) in favor of ATCs [23]. The evidence supporting the inclusion of physician extenders in the orthopedic practice as a means of generating revenue is abundant.

The most traditional means by which mid-level practitioners are utilized to help the bottom line in an orthopedic practice is through billing for patient services rendered in clinic and via surgical assistant fees in the operating room. In a 2010 article, physician assistants were even named as the sixth best "ancillary service to increase your orthopedic practice revenue," following more traditional ancillaries on the list such as physical therapy, advanced imaging services, DME programs, electromyography, and surgery centers. While not conventionally viewed as an "ancillary service," the article cited that practices employing PAs to both see patients and assist in the O.R. commonly generated 2–3x the PAs salary in revenue [24].

Keeping Everyone Happy

Neither party in the physician–mid-level relationship will be content for very long if the hiring MD's principal objectives are not being met. If the chief goal in incorporating an MLP was to create a more efficient system and reduce overall time in the office, then an increase in patient volume and upswing in practice revenue will not matter as much if the clinic days remain long. The appropriate system needs to be installed so that the ATC, NP, or PA is utilized in order to meet the foremost goals of the supervising physician and their practice ideals.

In a recent survey of the Physician Assistants in Orthopedic Surgery (PAOS), 91% of respondents noted being "satisfied" or "very satisfied" with their position as a full-time PA practicing in orthopedic surgery [12]. 75% of this group of orthopedic PAs reported working an average of 50 or less hours weekly (not including call), and 96% reported 60 or less hours weekly [12]. There are, of course, numerous ways to help avoid clinician burnout in the orthopedic practice, but certainly keeping average weekly workload to a mean of less than 50 h is a good start.

In 2016, the mean full-time base salary for nurse practitioners in all specialties was $102,526 [3]. The 2016 survey data of PAOS conveys a mean base salary of $110,550 with an average total annual compensation of nearly $125,000 [12]. This same group of PAs reports an average of 24 days paid time off annually, attributing 19 of those to personal vacation time and 5 to continuing education time [12]. The average reported allowance for CME annually was $2150 (range 0–$7500). 62% of the orthopedic surgery PAs reported receiving a financial bonus, with an average reported bonus of $15,995 [12].

The combination of reasonable work–life balance, potential for tremendous autonomy, broad scope of practice, and comfortable income capability explain why the most recent offering of US News & World Report's "100 Best Jobs" list nurse practitioners and physician assistants at #2 and #3, respectively [25].

Aside from the traditional focuses of finances and work hours, there will exist a certain subset of intangibles that will carry the potential to add exponential value to the job, both on the physician's side and the clinician's and administrative/support staff side. This refers to each team member's unique recipe for motivation and what drives them. What makes them tick? For some clinicians or team members, this altruistic "bonus" may come in the form of a quarterly happy hour or a community team-building event. For others, it may be the ability to maintain protected time off for travel, or some intermittent flex time for morning exercise. Some mid-level practitioners will value the opportunity to offload the physician's academic or community speaking engagements. Others might relish more the chance at learning a new skill semi-autonomously, such as harvesting a graft or performing office ultrasound. Regardless, the supervising physician that can successfully tap into their staff's individual and collective passions will succeed in ways other practices can only imagine. Simply stated, the ability to build a team out of the orthopedic practice that harnesses the best of each member's abilities in this way will determine whether the clinicians involved view their position as "just a job in ortho" versus an "orthopedic career."

Future Visions/Conclusion

At a time when healthcare reform is driving the movement for improved access to care, cost-effective treatments, improved documentation and increased efforts at health maintenance and prevention, mid-level providers offer a formidable option to partner with physicians more than ever. In nearly countless ways, it is evident that incorporating athletic trainers, nurse practitioners, or physician assistants into the orthopedic practice can not only improve patient satisfaction, outcomes, and compliance but also increase practice efficiency, revenue, and expand reach all in a safe and cost-effective manner. The evidence suggests that unless PAs and NPs are empowered to deliver care to the greatest possible allowance of their license, it is difficult to maximize their value. Most importantly, the development and refining of organizational culture regarding the value of mid-level practitioners is paramount in impacting their utilization. With the right amount of planning, proper communication, and some good fortune in harnessing the team's collective energy, the incorporation of mid-level providers can predictably bring synergy to the orthopedic practice.

Author's Disclaimer For purposes of this chapter, the term "mid-level practitioner" (MLP) will be utilized to loosely bundle the "nonphysician" group of advanced practice providers and clinicians entailing nurse practitioners (NPs), physician assistants (PAs), certified athletic trainers (ATCs), and other physician extenders such as nurse midwives, nurse anesthetists, and physical therapists.

References

1. Marjoua Y, Bozic KJ. Brief history of quality movement in US healthcare. Curr Rev Musculoskelet Med. 2012;5(4):265–73.
2. PAs Practice Medicine. American Academy of PAs 2017. 2017.
3. Jennings N, Lee G, Chao K, Keating S. A survey of patient satisfaction in a metropolitan emergency department: comparing nurse practitioners and emergency physicians. Int J Nurs Pract. 2009;15(3):213–8.
4. Katz JA. The evolving role of PAs: American Academy of PAs; 2016.
5. A look at each APRN role. HealthCom, Media. 2017
6. Glotzbecker BE, Yolin-Raley DS, DeAngelo DJ, Stone RM, Soiffer RJ, Alyea EP. Impact of physician assistants on the outcomes of patients with acute myelogenous leukemia receiving chemotherapy in an Academic Medical Center. J Oncol Pract. 2013;9(5):e228–33.
7. The Connecticut Academy of Physician Assistants Government Affairs Committee. ConnAPA scope of practice request. Connecticut academy of physician assistants. 2017.
8. Furlow B. Nurse practitioners outscore physicians in patient satisfaction survey: Haymarket Media, Inc; 2011.
9. Brady MI. A survey assessing patient satisfaction with physician assistant care at the maple street clinic. School of Physician Assistant Studies. 2004;127:1–29.
10. Zerehi MR, Rathfon E. Internists and physician assistants: team-based primary care: American College of Physicians; 2010.
11. Medical Group Management Association. Physician compensation and production survey: 2009 report based on 2008 data. Englewood: Co: Medical Group Management Association; 2009. p. 2009.
12. 2016 Practice and Salary Survey Report. Physician assistants Orthopaedic surgery. 2016.
13. Program Outcomes. Commission on accreditation of athletic training education. 2018.
14. NCCPA. Exam development and scoring. 2018.
15. Larson EH, Coerver DA, Wick KH, Ballweg RA. Physician assistants in orthopedic practice. A national study. J Allied Health. 2011;40(4):174–80.
16. State of California. Frequently asked questions about supervising physician assistants. 2016 state of California. 2016.
17. Scope of practice FAQs for consumers. National Council of state boards of nursing. 2018.
18. Smith T. Athletic trainers pump up Care in Orthopedics Clinic. UCHealth Central Insider. 2015;8(18)
19. Larkin GL, Hooker RS. Patient willingness to be seen by physician assistants, nurse practitioners, and residents in the emergency department: does the presumption of assent have an empirical basis? Am J Bioeth. 2010;10(8):1–10.
20. Hiring a PA: the benefits for physicians and practices. American Academy of physician assistants. 2004.
21. DeCapua M. How much revenue does a primary care nurse practitioner generate? Barton Associates; 2016.
22. Liu N, Finkelstein SR, Poghosyan L. A new model for nurse practitioner utilization in primary care: increased efficiency and implications. Health Care Manag Rev. 2014;39(1):10–20.
23. Pecha FQ, Xerogeanes JW, Karas SG, Himes ME, Mines BA. Comparison of the effect of medical assistants versus certified athletic trainers on patient volumes and revenue generation in a sports medicine practice. Sports Health. 2013;5(4):337–9.
24. Dunn L. 6 Ancillary services to increase your orthopedic practice revenue: ASC Communications; 2010.
25. U.S. News & World Report Announces the 2017 Best Jobs. U.S. News & World Report LP. 2017.

Chapter 5
Social Media Use in the Field of Orthopedic Surgery

Mohsin S. Fidai, Joseph S. Tramer, Toufic R. Jildeh, Sasha Stine, Fabien Meta, and Eric C. Makhni

Introduction

Over the past few decades, the Internet has transformed the landscape of healthcare, particularly with the advent of social media and social networking. In 2017 there were over 1 billion Facebook users and 500 million Twitter users, with 80% of Americans utilizing some form of social media. (https://www.statista.com/statistics/273476/percentage-of-us-population-with-a-social-network-profile/) [1]. There are an estimated 6.5 million health-related search queries per day, and patients are using the Internet as a primary resource when managing their health [2]. Over 70% of Internet users state that they have accessed health information online [3]. The integration of social media into everyday life has made platforms such as Facebook, Twitter, YouTube, and Instagram increasingly important tools for patient-physician interaction. Demographic studies have shown that while there is a significant difference in age and gender, with an increased number of young and female users, there is a fairly equal distribution across education, income, race/ethnicity, and rural and urban locations of social media participants [4]. This highlights social media's potential for outreach to a multitude of patient populations.

M. S. Fidai (✉) · J. S. Tramer · T. R. Jildeh
Henry Ford Health System, Department of Orthopedic Surgery, Detroit, MI, USA
e-mail: mfidai1@hfhs.org; jtramer1@hfhs.org; tjildeh1@hfhs.org

S. Stine · F. Meta
Wayne State University School of Medicine, Henry Ford Hospital, Department of Orthopedic Surgery, Detroit, MI, USA
e-mail: sstin@med.wayne.edu; fmeta@med.wayne.edu

E. C. Makhni
Division of Sports Medicine, Department of Orthopedic Surgery, Henry Ford Health System, West Bloomfield, MI, USA

E. C. Makhni et al. (eds.), *Orthopedic Practice Management*,
https://doi.org/10.1007/978-3-319-96938-1_5

Recent literature has evaluated the use of social media among patients and providers [5–7]. A 2013 systematic review identified seven key uses of social media for health communication:

1. Provide health information on a range of conditions
2. Provide answers to medical questions
3. Facilitate dialogue patient-to-patient and patient-to-health professional
4. Collect data on patient experiences and opinions
5. Health intervention, health promotion, and health education
6. Reduce illness stigma
7. Provide online consultations [8]

This study, and others, demonstrates the increased use of social media not only as a means for researching medical maladies and conditions but also for physician selection. Websites such as HealthGrades.com, rateMD.com, and vitals.com make searching and comparing physician reviews quick and easy for patients. With an increasingly competitive marketplace for orthopedic surgeons, patient recruitment has become a primary barrier to practice advancement. The purpose of this chapter is to analyze how both patients and physicians interact with social media, and to outline future steps providers can take to integrate social media into their practices.

Patients on Social Media

The Patient Experience on Social Media

Patients primarily use social media to increase knowledge regarding medical conditions or ailments, exchange advice with fellow patients or providers and for social support [9]. A study conducted in 2016 observed how patients utilized Instagram in their postoperative period following ACL surgery. Using the hashtag #aclsurgery, the investigators characterized the ways in which patients used social media to outline their experiences with surgery. It was found that the majority of posts were personal recovery stories, with over 90% of posts including postoperative photographs [10]. Other significant mentions included messages regarding progress with postoperative rehabilitation and return to sport. In just 1 year there were almost 1000 Instagram posts related to scoliosis in the adolescent population. These individuals used social media as a platform for sharing progress stories and photos, while providing support and motivation for other patients with similar conditions [11]. Patients have also shared their experiences online following total joint arthroplasty. In a query of Instagram hashtags, it was found that total knee patients were likely to share stories on the rehabilitation process and wound healing, while total hip patients posted about their return to activities of daily living [12]. Multiple studies have reiterated the findings in the previously detailed investigations, showing that most patient interactions on social media highlight progress in wound healing, rehabilitation, and activities of daily living. This provides unique insight into patients' priorities during treatment and allows orthopedic surgeons to better understand postoperative patient expectations.

Patients are also likely to utilize social media to find support from others facing similar obstacles. Individuals receiving diagnoses that no one in their immediate offline network has experienced can be isolating. Websites such as patientslikeme.com provide a platform for information and story sharing between people with similar health problems. These have the benefit of providing support for patients undergoing similar trials and tribulations but offer the potential downfall of receiving advice from unqualified sources [13].

Physician Review Websites

A study in 2014 found that 47% of patients have searched for health providers online and 37% have consulted a physician rating website before seeking care [14]. These numbers will only increase as a younger generation of patients begins using the Internet to help choose between the many available providers. Websites such as Healthgrades.com, RateMDs.com, Vitals.com, and Yelp.com provide platforms for patients to grade physicians and leave comments regarding their care experiences and perceptions. The measures used for grading vary between websites, but overall they tend to encompass the entirety of the patient experience. A review of over 2000 patient ratings of orthopedic surgeons showed that high scores in five variables were statistically significant for higher ratings including ease of scheduling, time spent with the patient, wait time, surgeon proficiency, and bedside manner [15]. However, many websites ask about interactions with office staff and the cleanliness or appearance of the clinic in addition to perceptions of the physician and the quality of care delivered. Frost et al. found that over 90% of orthopedic surgeons have at least one review online, but many only have a handful of reviews [14]. Those with a small sample size can suffer with just one negative review. Thus, it is important to be cognizant of online grades and address any complaints that have been brought up on the review sites.

YouTube

YouTube is the second most utilized search engine behind Google. There are millions of videos posted yearly on the website, including an abundance of healthcare-related content. Simply searching "total knee replacement" on YouTube yields over 200,000 results. Online videos can be a useful tool for reaching patients and provide an opportunity to further educate patients on their conditions. A recent study demonstrated the far reach of YouTube videos, with over 65,000 views in 1 year on their informational video on vaccinations [16]. The Mayo clinic provided a set of

YouTube videos to patients prior to hip and knee replacement. The videos were created as a "virtual hospital experience" in order to give patients a preview of what to expect during their stay. They found that the study arm randomized to watch videos beforehand had lower anxiety scores and felt more comfortable with their upcoming surgery [17]. Many patients watch videos of their surgery beforehand, which can lead to both reassurance and increased anxiety.

Physicians on Social Media

The Physician Experience

With the overwhelming majority of patients using social media for both personal and health-related purposes, an Internet presence by the physician has become increasingly important. A recent survey showed that while 90% of doctors use social media for personal use, only 65% use these platforms for professional reasons [18]. Physicians are primarily using social media in order to better communicate with colleagues and for marketing purposes, rather than patient engagement [9]. Studies investigating the habits of physicians interacting on social media show the majority of its use is to network with other healthcare professionals, share research, discuss challenging cases, and engage in health advocacy [19]. An underwhelming minority are actually using social media to engage with patients [20]. While surgeons have a strong presence on LinkedIn, which can be used to collaborate with colleagues and display professional accolades, there is a lower presence on platforms such as Instagram and Twitter [11]. A survey of 321 orthopedic surgeons, from a variety of practice settings, showed that surgeons in the private sector, rather than academic, were significantly more likely to engage patients online [21]. This represents a disconnect between patients and providers but also represents an important opportunity for practice development.

Professional Networking and Education

There are a multitude of websites and forums for orthopedic surgeons to network, share ideas, and discuss cases. With continual advancement in online live video streaming, a number of websites have begun broadcasting everything from lectures to live OR feeds. Orthogate.com, orlive.com, vumedi.com are examples of commonly used websites for physician education. The incredible advances of live video allow surgeons to communicate face to face over any distance and demonstrate techniques to doctors across the globe. In addition to lectures and other educational materials, these websites host open forums that encourage discussion between providers on topics ranging from difficult cases to practice management.

Another social media network involving many orthopedic surgeons is researchgate.com. This website allows members to create a profile linked to their academic research and publications. By viewing a profile one is able to see the projects being worked on by that individual and request access to previous publications. Additionally, the website provides areas to allow discussion of scientific articles and current research topics. With the vast amount of research continuously conducted throughout the world, this can be an invaluable resource to connect with investigators everywhere.

Practice Promotion

As mentioned throughout this chapter, your patients are more likely than not to be interacting on social media on a daily basis. Millions of Americans use social media for a number of reasons, but only 5% have interacted with a health professional online [22]. This represents a huge number of individuals that can be reached via social media. While physicians are using social media to connect with one another, there is an underwhelming amount of patient outreach on these platforms. A recent study showed that 57% of consumers state a hospital's social media presence influenced their choice on where to go for services and over 80% stated engaging in social media gave the perception that the hospital was technologically advanced [18]. Dr. Howard Luks, in a 2012 AAOS publication, stated that his strong online presence has contributed to gaining up to ten additional new patient inquiries a day [23]. Particularly as younger generations begin requiring orthopedic care, social media will become an increasingly important platform for patient outreach and communication.

Blogs

Since the early 1990s, the Internet was reformatted to Web 2.0, a platform that allowed users to generate their own content to post online for consumption. This opened the door for blogging, a website in which the user posts content that is freely available to read online. According to a report by the Pew Internet and American Life Project (Pew), 8% (12 million) of 147 million adult users of the Internet in the United States keep a blog, while 39% (57 million) read one. http://www.pewinternet.org/2015/10/08/social-networking-usage-2005-2015/ [24]. Over the past decade, there have been a number of peer-reviewed studies demonstrating the effectiveness of blogs in disseminating health-related information, engaging patients and for professional development [25–27]. A survey conducted on medical bloggers found that successful writers with large followings tended to be highly educated writers and provided sources along with practical knowledge to their readers [28]. Healthcare institutions such as the Mayo clinic have utilized blogs to foster discussion among patients and providers. Online blogs can be used to advertise facilities, allow patients to share positive experiences, and feature prominent physicians. Individual physicians have used blogs to discuss current problems in healthcare, address frequently asked questions, and outline treatment protocols for patients. Additionally, blogs can be used to discuss scientific research and to help recruit patients to participate in clinical studies [29].

Blogs also provide patients a platform to discuss their ailments and share their experiences. There are numerous blogs discussing living with chronic conditions such as diabetes or coping with a cancer diagnosis and treatment. These can provide patients with a safe place to discuss health-related issues with other patients and draw from their experiences.

Wikipedias

Wikis are collaborative websites that allow users to add, edit, and delete content freely. The most popular wiki, Wikipedia, is a free online encyclopedia that encompasses thousands of topics. Medicine is a commonly researched topic on Wikipedia, with the top 200 medical articles receiving over 100,000 monthly views [30]. There are also individual wikis dedicated to subtopics including one for Orthopedic Surgery. These are commonly used resources by both patients and providers as they provide quick and easily accessible information. Many are wary of these sources due to the ability of public users to edit and change information, however, these websites are typically well policed for false information. A study comparing Wikipedia drug pages to their corresponding Medscape Drug Reference pages found that it included roughly 76% of the same information with most differences due to omission rather than false information [31]. While these websites can provide an initial source of information, it is important to understand their limitations and educate patients on this reality.

Physician Websites

Physician websites serve as a platform for patients to access information about the physician and the practice. A professional website is often the first impression patients have of you. Maintaining an up-to-date and well-organized website will leave the impression that your practice is the same.

Professional website domain names should be simple and easy to remember. Many physician website domain names are simply the physician's first and last names followed their professional degrees (i.e., JohnSmithMD.com). The website should be user-friendly and easy to navigate. The homepage should offer links for patients to access information about the physician, the practice, educational resources, and contact information. Avoid using overly technical terminology and medical jargon. The website can serve to educate patients about their conditions as well as prepare them for their clinic visit. Websites can offer methods for patients to make appointments online. They can streamline the new patient experience by providing forms online so patients can fill them out prior to their clinic visit. Many surgeons also have their preoperative and postoperative protocols available on their website for easy accessibility for patients and physical therapists.

The website can serve as a method of consolidating your online persona. Links to profession Instagram, Facebook, Twitter, and other social media outlets should be easily accessible on the homepage. Links to your professional website can be placed on your social media accounts to increase traffic to your website. Additionally, the website should be mobile friendly to allow patients to seamlessly access the content on their mobile devices.

One hurdle that many physicians encounter is how to actually get a web page up and running. There are many "DIY" solutions using platforms such as WordPress, but most physicians find it easiest to contract with a company or web design specialist to build the page for them. Regardless of how the page is built, the physician should try to perform SEO, or search engine optimization. This is a strategy that incorporates keywords, updates, and novel content into the website so that the page can be found more easily during web searches, especially within a particular geography and topic (e.g. "sports medicine + Detroit metro"). Therefore, having a web page is one thing, but keeping it actively updated and current is an additional investment that will help attract patients (and new patients) to your page.

Misinformation and Social Media

While the advancement of the Internet and social media has provided an incredible wealth of information for both patient and providers, this has unfortunately opened the door for the spread of misinformation. There are a plethora of studies demonstrating the amount of low-quality information available on the Internet [32, 33]. Eighty-five percent of physicians have reported experiencing a patient bringing information from the Internet to a visit [6]. Doctors are often using clinic time to answer questions based Internet articles with little to no scientific merit, including defending diagnoses that may run contrary to what patients have read online [34]. A study searching social media for mentions of cellular therapy injections for the treatment of musculoskeletal conditions found a wide range of advertisements and statements from drug companies on this therapy. An overwhelming majority of the statements were positive and did not highlight the risks, benefits, and limitations of a largely unproven therapy [35]. Physicians frequently receive questions from patients regarding therapies or treatment modalities seen advertised online. It is important to be aware of these messages and educate patients using evidence-based information.

Important Considerations Before Using Social Media

A review in 2014 outlined principles for physicians participating in social media [29]. The first and most important principle requires maintenance of professionalism. Institutions typically issue guidelines regarding social media use; it is important to be aware and follow these mandates. A social media presence must begin with a set of policies that respect legal and regulatory limits consistent with your individual organization. Setting out guidelines is an important step in ensuring posts are consistent with organizational policies, without requiring constant monitoring, and approval for posting online. Confidentiality remains vital during social media interaction and HIPPA guidelines must be followed online. It is imperative to get expressed permission from patients before any online interaction. It is also important to recognize that while messages over social media may be private, they are often not secure exchanges of information. If there is any doubt as to the appropriateness of a post, it should not be shared.

Getting Started on Social Media

An article published on AAOS Now outlined a few tips for getting started by Dr. Howard Luks, an orthopedic surgeon, who has successfully developed an online presence. He starts by defining an objective. Social media encompasses many facets from blogs and tweets to videos and Facebook pages, and it is important to define your goal as an online presence. Additionally, it is important to define your persona. Be consistent with your message and remain genuine while participating in social media. It is important to engage the audience regularly in order to keep content fresh and encourage participation. Be realistic about reaching your goals. Creating a social media account will not cause an influx of patients overnight and developing a following takes time and patience. It is important for any physician to include a disclaimer including your right to remove content and also that engagement over social media channels does not represent a true doctor-patient relationship. Additionally, by setting up a simple Google alert, it is easy to monitor what patients are saying about you and your social media presence in order to continuously improve and adapt. Finally, engaging with other healthcare professionals who have successfully incorporated social media into their practice is an invaluable resource when getting started [36].

References

1. Statista: The Statistics Portal. Percentage of U.S. population with a social media profile from 2008 to 2017. (https://www.statista.com/statistics/273476/percentage-of-us-population-with-a-social-network-profile/).

2. Sculco PK, McLawhorn AS, Fehring KA, De Martino I. The future of social media in orthopedic surgery. Curr Rev Musculoskelet Med. 2017;10(2):278–9.
3. Campbell L, Evans Y, Pumper M, Moreno MA. Social media use by physicians: a qualitative study of the new frontier of medicine. BMC Med Inform Decis Mak. 2016;16:91.
4. Thackeray R, Crookston BT, West JH. Correlates of health-related social media use among adults. J Med Internet Res. 2013;15(1):e21.
5. Barry F. Social media 101 for health care development organizations. AHP J. 2010;30–4.
6. Danquah G, Mittal V, Solh M, Kolachalam RB. Effect of internet use on patient's surgical outcomes. Int Surg. 2007;92(6):339–43.
7. Patel R, Chang T, Greysen SR, Chopra V. Social media use in chronic disease: a systematic review and novel taxonomy. Am J Med. 2015 Dec;128(12):1335–50.
8. Moorhead SA, Hazlett DE, Harrison L, Carroll JK, Irwin A, Hoving C. A new dimension of health care: systematic review of the uses, benefits, and limitations of social media for health communication. J Med Internet Res. 2013 Apr;15(4):e85.
9. Antheunis ML1, Tates K, Nieboer TE. Patients' and health professionals' use of social media in health care: motives, barriers and expectations. Patient Educ Couns. 2013;92(3):426–31.
10. Ramkumar PN, La T Jr, Fisch E, Fabricant PD, White AE, Jones KJ, Taylor SA. Integrating social media and anterior cruciate ligament surgery: an analysis of patient, surgeon, and hospital use. Arthroscopy. 2017 Mar;33(3):579–85.
11. Haeberle HS, Egger AC, Navarro SM, Cornaghie MM, Ramkumar PN, Goodwin RC, Mont MA. Social media and pediatric scoliosis: an analysis of patient and surgeon use. Surg Technol Int. 2017 Oct 12;31:189–96.
12. Ramkumar PN, Navarro SM, Haeberle HS, Chughtai M, Flynn ME, Mont MA. Social media and Total joint arthroplasty: an analysis of patient utilization on Instagram. J Arthroplast. 2017 Sep;32(9):2694–700.
13. Rupert DJ, Moultrie RR, Read JG, Amoozegar JB, Bornkessel AS, O'Donoghue AC, Sullivan HW. Perceived healthcare provider reactions to patient and caregiver use of online health communities. Patient Educ Couns. 2014;96(3):320–6.
14. Frost C, Mesfin A. Online reviews of orthopedic surgeons: an emerging trend. Orthopedics. 2015;38(4):e257–62.
15. Bakhsh W, Mesfin A. Online ratings of orthopedic surgeons: analysis of 2185 reviews. Am J Orthop (Belle Mead NJ). 2014;43(8):359–63.
16. Harrison D, Wilding J, Bowman A, Fuller A, Nicholls SG, Pound CM, et al. Using YouTube to disseminate effective vaccination pain treatment for babies. PLoS One 2016;11(10):e0164123.
17. O'Connor MI, Brennan K, Kazmerchak S, Pratt J. YouTube videos to create a "virtual hospital experience" for hip and knee replacement patients to decrease preoperative anxiety: a randomized trial. Interact J Med Res. 2016;5(2):e10.
18. Ventola CL. Social media and health care professionals: benefits, risks, and best practices. P T. 2014 Jul;39(7):491–499, 520.
19. Fogelson NS, Rubin ZA, Ault KA. Beyond likes and tweets: an in-depth look at the physician social media landscape. Clin Obstet Gynecol. 2013 Sep;56(3):495–508.
20. Chretien KC, Kind T. Social media and clinical care: ethical, professional, and social implications. Circulation. 2013;127(13):1413–21.
21. Duymuş TM, Karadeniz H, Şükür E, Atiç R, Zehir S, Azboy İ. Social media and internet usage of orthopaedic surgeons. J Clin Orthop Trauma. 2017 Jan-Mar;8(1):25–30.
22. McLawhorn AS, De Martino I, Fehring KA, Sculco PK. Social media and your practice: navigating the surgeon-patient relationship. Curr Rev Musculoskelet Med. 2016;9(4):487–95.
23. Luks H. Chapter 3/establishing a digital presence. In: Soyer A, editor. American Academy of Orthopaedic surgeons. AAOS practice management committee. Rosemont: Social Media in Healthcare: A Primer for Orthopaedic Surgeons; 2012.
24. Perrin A. Social media usage: 2005–2015. Pew internet and American life project (pew). http://www.pewinternet.org/2015/10/08/social-networking-usage-2005-2015/.
25. Kennedy RS. Weblogs, social software, and new interactivity on the web. Psychiatr Serv. 2004 Mar;55(3):247–9.

26. Price B. Disseminating best practice through a web log. Nurs Stand. 2010;24(29):35–40.
27. Carley S, Beardsell I, May N, Crowe L, Baombe J, Grayson A, et al. Social-media-enabled learning in emergency medicine: a case study of the growth, engagement and impact of a free open access medical education blog. Postgrad med J Postgrad Med J 2018;94(1108):92–96.
28. Kovic I, Lulic I, Brumini G. Examining the medical blogosphere: an online survey of medical bloggers. J Med Internet Res. 2008 Sep 23;10(3):e28.
29. Grajales FJ 3rd, Sheps S, Ho K, Novak-Lauscher H, Eysenbach G. Social media: a review and tutorial of applications in medicine and health care. J Med Internet Res. 2014;16(2):e13.
30. Heilman JM, Kemmann E, Bonert M, Chatterjee A, Ragar B, Beards GM, et al. Wikipedia: a key tool for global public health promotion. J Med Internet Res. 2011;13(1):e14.
31. Clauson KA, Polen HH, Boulos MN, Dzenowagis JH. Scope, completeness, and accuracy of drug information in Wikipedia. Ann Pharmacother. 2008;42(12):1814–21.
32. Garcia GH, Taylor SA, Dy CJ, Christ A, Patel RM, Dines JS. Online resources for shoulder instability: what are patients reading? J Bone Joint Surg Am. 2014 Oct 15;96(20):e177.
33. Fabricant PD, Dy CJ, Patel RM, Blanco JS, Doyle SM. Internet search term affects the quality and accuracy of online information about developmental hip dysplasia. J Pediatr Orthop. 2013 Jun;33(4):361–5.
34. Ahmad F, Hudak PL, Bercovitz K, Hollenberg E, Levinson W. Are physicians ready for patients with internet-based health information? J Med Internet Res. 2006 Sep 29;8(3):e22.
35. Ramkumar PN, Navarro SM, Haeberle HS, Chughtai M, Demetriades C, Piuzzi NS, et al. Cellular therapy injections in today's orthopedic market: a social media analysis. Cytotherapy. 2017;19(12):1392–9.
36. Schafer MF, Pearson LL. Social media for orthopaedic surgeons. AAOS now. 2010 October. https://www.aaos.org/AAOSNow/2010/Oct/youraaos/youraaos11/?ssopc=1.

Part II
Leadership and Management

Chapter 6
Building and Managing a Successful Private Practice

Joseph M. Lombardi, Melvin C. Makhni, and Joseph S. Lombardi

Benefits of Private Practice

There are multiple benefits to running a private practice, but the most profound continues to be the autonomy provided to the surgeon in nearly all aspects of the practice. This includes maintaining control over operational decisions, revenue streams, patient care, advertising, and marketing. Physicians operating in a private practice can set their own schedules, decide what days to work and when to take vacation. This contrasts to hospital employment structures, which often control the work hours, vacation days, and number of patients that must been seen. Private practice also affords the practitioner greater control over personnel, allowing for hiring or firing of employees to meet the needs of a constantly evolving practice. Furthermore, private practices offer financial and employment stability that is not found in a hospital employment model. For example, a practitioner in a private model can control their revenue streams. This includes increasing the number of patients that are seen as well as utilization of ancillary services, i.e., physical therapy, imaging, bracing, and ambulatory surgery centers that are not available as revenue sources under an employment model. These can be substantial sources of additional income for the private practitioner. While some salary models may provide bonuses for performance benchmarks, many remain a flat salary, hampering a

J. M. Lombardi (✉)
Orthopedic Surgery, Columbia University Medical Center, Department of Orthopedic Surgery, New York, NY, USA

M. C. Makhni
Brigham and Women's Hospital, Harvard Medical School, Department of Orthopedic Surgery, Boston, MA, USA

J. S. Lombardi
JFK Medical Center, Edison Surgical Center, Department of Orthopedic Surgery, Edison, NJ, USA

E. C. Makhni et al. (eds.), *Orthopedic Practice Management*,
https://doi.org/10.1007/978-3-319-96938-1_6

physician's ability to increase revenue. Lastly, while contracts offered by hospitals may be enticing initially, they may be subject to unfavorable renegotiation or even termination by the hospital employer which leaves the physician with little bargaining power. All of these factors contribute to private practice offering greater security and autonomy than other current practice models.

Deciding to Enter Private Practice

Private practice comes with several benefits, but it is not for everyone. Understanding yourself, your goals, and your priorities is the first step. Before entering private practice, you have to make a commitment that you want to be involved in running a practice. If you want to just practice your craft without thinking about billing, changing legislation, meaningful use, PQRS, and all the other headaches of the changing medical climate, then private practice is not for you. Whether you are a partner in a firm, or are the one managing the practice, all of those events will continue to happen, and only those groups who are forward-looking and actively adapting will be able to survive and thrive through the continuous challenges.

You should be interested in spending your time focusing on the clinical aspects of your practice, but you also should be willing to at least understand all the other components of the practice. Especially as a leader in a group, you have to know how to do every job. You can hire workers and managers as necessary, and it is important to trust them; but, if they tell you that a job takes a certain length of time or that it cannot be done, you have to know that to be true. You cannot, for example, purchase an EMR system and ask your staff to figure it out – you have to be part of the process, learning the ins and outs of the system. If you do not have the knowledge to check on those working for you, you will not be able to run your practice efficiently and cost-effectively.

Some private practices are integrated with residents and fellows, so a teaching atmosphere can be possible. More possible is the ability to "be academic." The distinction no longer exists between "academic" and "private" practices, as the lines have continued to blur, with some private practices giving salaries, and many academic institutions moving toward RVU or production-based compensation. Being academic involves studying protocols and analyzing outcomes, and constantly striving to improve processes and techniques. This can arguably be done better in a private practice setting in which you have much more control over the system you practice in, and several private practice groups around the country have been examples in showing this to be the case.

While it may seem daunting to tackle all the business challenges that we are never taught during medical school, do not be afraid to enter into private practice, even as an independent practitioner. If you are good at your specialty and willing to work hard and learn, then you will be fine. Do not worry about the competition in the area; competitive environments will simply require you to be more aggressive in making contacts in the area and taking other steps to build your practice base.

It takes years sometimes to build up a successful referral practice. Hard work is one of the most important ingredients to developing a practice. If you are focused solely on your specialty of interest, it can be more difficult to build up patient volume. You will get more referrals if you are available to patients and other physicians and simply kind to them, everywhere from the emergency room to the routine office setting. Taking ER calls, living close to the hospital, and being good to the ER and hospital staff goes a long way in the relationship building that helps jumpstart practices. You might be surprised how many physicians might refer to you if you ask them to. They were all there at the early stages themselves at one time, so many of them like helping the younger doctors get onto their feet.

Also, do not be afraid to take the financial risk. There are countless "safer" options where you can get a guaranteed salary and steady practice, but those come with restrictions and dependency on your employers as well. Banks will give low-interest loans to young physicians, so you will be able to acquire the necessary financing for your office and other expenses. It is not uncommon at the start of practice to have a home office or work out of the office of a colleague. Then, once you get an office, you may not have the frills of other more established colleagues, as you will have to do whatever necessary to minimize unnecessary costs.

Components of a Practice

There are several essential components of any successful private practice. Each practice, in addition to the orthopedic surgeon, must have billing, front desk, and medical assistant personnel. Starting a practice, a surgeon must be aware that each physician will need about three staff members to support each of them. As practices grow, this ratio can actually increase from 3:1 to 5:1 as operations become more complex and ancillary services are incorporated.

Front Desk

Your front desk personnel are extremely important. They are the first contact a patient has in your office and a representative of you and your practice. Patients have said in the past that they love a certain doctor but would not go back to that person because they had such an unpleasant experience with the front desk employee.

Multiple factors make an excellent front desk staff – the most important which is pleasantness. They must be able to greet people well and make all patients feel respected, even when patients are waiting for their appointments, or if they are already unhappy with a complication from surgery. It is also helpful for them to be meticulous. They are charged with making the appropriate scheduling decisions, so they should be well versed in how to make appointments and independently make thoughtful decisions in unclear situations, and when to involve the medical assistant or the physician in unclear circumstances.

They should also be vigilant with collecting fees. It is not an easy skill to be pleasant and accommodating to patients, but also insistent in collecting co-pays. Sometimes patients arrive without their co-pays; at the end of a year in a multi-physician group, those missed payments can easily add up to tens of thousands of dollars in lost earnings, which will then require paying hourly wages to personnel to individually collect those co-pays – it simply is not cost effective. So, a system must be in place and adhered to; we prefer to collect co-payments before the patient visit begins, and if necessary refund co-payments if insurance plans dictate such. Patients who do not have cash or check with them should be offered the option to pay with credit card. Some patients who do not bring payment and refuse to pay, despite it being written on their insurance cards that there is a co-payment, may have no intention of paying for service at all. So, those patients must be treated respectfully by the front desk staff, but also with vigilance to collect payments to avoid significant losses to the practice.

Billing

Billing can be done in-house or outsourced. The benefits of having billing under the roof of the practice is that you have direct contact with the billing team and can collaborate with and oversee them very easily. And, it is easier to train and customize their services when they are in-house, so you may get better service from your own team – especially if you have a good manager of your billing department. Having your own billing personnel may cost more, however. For the smaller groups or independent practitioner, outsourced billing may be more cost-effective, but it is imperative that they are closely monitored – billing mistakes happen, and may happen at a higher rate in an outsourced model. And it is important to remember when mistakes happen, they are often to the loss of the physician. Payroll services like ADP are helpful as the billing department grows, and they can incorporate services such as direct deposit. Again though, services like these also make mistakes, so it is imperative that someone from your practice monitors them. A full-time accountant can be an asset in middle and larger sized practices to monitor the practice's finances. Regardless of your billing setup, hiring an outside independent billing company to review your procedures may help you identify suboptimal areas of your financial setup.

Medical Assistants

A medical assistant should be incorporated immediately into a physician's workflow. One of the biggest problems we have today in medicine (and orthopedic surgery is no different) is the amount of paperwork that we do. A medical assistant is necessary to help with patient flow in the office. The surgeon should devote as much time to direct patient care as possible, so assistants can help in countless ways; for example, if an MRI is denied, assistants can help with the paperwork and appeal letters, and follow-up with the insurance company and the patient is required to ensure proper care for the patient.

Once one gets sufficiently busy, a surgeon can consider hiring a physician assistant or nurse practitioner. This comes at a significant expense, so should be done when a surgeon thinks that patients seen and surgeries scheduled can increase by an amount that will more than offset the salary of the assistant. Not only can having an NP or PA help with the throughput of patients, but they can also be trained to see routine follow-ups, nonoperative patients, and spend more time with patients than the surgeon may be able to do alone in a busy practice. With the proper training by the surgeon, these practitioners can see these selected patients at a competency similar to the surgeon's, and should also be trained when to involve the surgeon if necessary. They can also help with surgeries and bill for their services as well.

Ancillaries

Ancillaries can be an important source of revenue, as well as serve as a convenient resource for your patients. Patients usually prefer to be able to get most of their needed service under one roof. For example, a patient with a compression fracture may follow up and need an X-ray, and after seeing you might need a brace. If they have to get their radiograph from one facility, and come see you, then you give a prescription for them to go pick up a brace somewhere else, it can be inconvenient, especially if your patient is an elderly patient in pain. Cost–benefit analysis should be performed looking at the resources you need to buy for the ancillary services as well as the employee salaries, and then understanding at what capacity you will be using those services to break even or make a profit.

Imaging

Being able to provide X-rays is convenient for not only patients but also for you. Patient flow is significantly improved as well, since patients who need radiographs will not always arrive to your facility after having had them, so they would need to leave to another facility, cancel their appointments, or have a less-than-optimal appointment, all of which clog up clinic time and decrease patient throughput. However, X-ray and a technician are considerable expenses and may not be necessary for smaller groups just starting out. The technician should be treated with ownership of the machine, since there will be times that the machine is down, or new parts need to be ordered. At least one physician partner in the group should also understand the machine so that you can work together if needed to get the machine back to function as expeditiously as possible in case of malfunction, to limit the disruption to patient flow and patient care that these situations will cause.

An MRI machine and technician is another considerable expense that can turn profit if your practice generates enough revenue from them. There are different costs of closed versus open, and differences in quality of MRI images that influence which machine is purchased. If needed, the MRI can be run in daytime hours or even be opened sometimes after-hours, if sufficiently busy.

Surgi-center

Your practice may want to own a surgi-center, or even join, buy into, or simply be affiliated with one. Ambulatory surgical centers are not as good of revenue streams as they were 10 years ago because now they are in network; more cases can now be done there but at lower reimbursements per case. Many practices who adamantly maintain their independence from hospitals also choose to affiliate their surgi-centers with hospitals. By doing so, the practice gets hospital reimbursements and as a by-product joins networks of all insurance companies. There can be a financial benefit in pricing and overhead by making this affiliation, but it is important to structure the agreement in a way that your practice still owns a majority stake in the facility and that you can continue to run your own practice independent of undue hospital regulation.

Bracing

The use of casts, splints, and bracing is an essential component in the nonoperative treatment of orthopedic conditions. Offering these services not only provides a convenience for your patient but an opportunity for a small source of revenue to the practitioner. Application of splints and casts can be billed for through Medicare or private insurers. Likewise, insurance reimbursement for bracing may allow for a small profit for the practice. Some insurance providers may have limitations to how many braces they will reimburse over a predetermined time period. It would be prudent to consult with the patient prior to prescribing a new brace as they may incur unexpected charges.

Physical Therapy

Physical therapy is another treatment modality commonly used for nonoperative and postoperative orthopedic conditions. Although revenues have seen a downward pressure over the past decade, this continues to provide the physician-owner with a steady source of income. Ownership should be considered on a case-by-case basis. If your group has enough referrals to open a physical therapy center, it may be beneficial to do so independently. Other options include buying into a therapy center with other physician-owners as a way to generate revenue.

Practice Structure

Practices should be structured to optimize revenue streams through two mechanisms: (1) maximize physician exposure to patients and (2) minimize overhead expenses. The evolution of ancillary staff in patient care has helped physicians to combat the increasingly cumbersome administrative burdens. For example, my practice utilizes NPs, PAs, and physiatrists in appropriate instances of initial consultation, longitudinal nonoperative management, and routine post-op visits. This allows the surgeons to focus their time on those patients who require surgical indications. Additionally, the utilization of nurses and scribes to help minimize the paperwork burden on the physician helps to maximize the number of patients that can be seen by the physician.

Running a private practice is akin to running a small business with some practices employing upwards of 50–100 staff members. While it is important for partners in the practice to understand the roles of each ancillary staff member, oftentimes the burden of running a practice is beyond the scope of the physician in terms of time and skill set. It is therefore vital to have a practice manager who can help to run the financial aspect of the practice. These managers often have advanced business or accounting degrees such as a MBA or CPA. It is their job to oversee the day-to-day operations of the practice including personnel management, scheduling, billing, and patient care satisfaction. This practice manager or COO will often work in conjunction with a managing partner to make small financial decisions, e.g., ordering a new printer. Major financial decisions are typically decided by vote among members of the practice. It is additionally the role of the practice manager to maximize profit by compiling routine quarterly financial reports which are then reviewed and analyzed by the partners. In large practice settings, it is also helpful to assign managers of each division. For example, by using a billing manager, scheduling manager, and front desk manager, there is a clear delineation of responsibility that helps to keep a practice overhead down. Marketing and advertisement are increasingly important as patients are more commonly relying on the Internet as a source of referral for new physicians. This can vary from having a simple website to advertising in local papers, magazines, or online. Finding a good marketing firm can be vital, especially for new practices. However, this is a process that should be discussed and agreed upon by all partners as it may represent a substantial upfront cost.

Tips for Maintaining a Practice

Fairness

A key to longevity in a practice is fairness. There is a lot of compromise that must occur on the parts of both senior and junior partners, and egos must be left at the door. It is unlikely that everyone will always agree, so it is important for the group to have a good working relationship and be able to compromise even when members of the group take unreasonable positions. Systems can be put in place to help ensure fairness, and it is important that no one, even the founding member, exerts their will over what is best for the group.

As an example, I started my practice many years ago and have expanded our group to have a dozen physicians and 60 total staff members. As the founding and senior member, I did not want to take calls. However, others also did not want to take calls so we voted in place a system in which I would no longer take calls at age 65. And, if I or anyone did not want to take calls, we would have to financially reimburse another member of the practice to take calls. The system was in place for quite some time, but then as more people came into the practice, the issue was revisited. Once this happened, a majority of partners did not feel that the age 65 calls provision was fair, so there was a new vote and the rule was overturned. Now, all partners including myself are responsible for taking calls or financially incentivizing others to do so, regardless of age. This is not in my best interest, and I could have stood firm with the initial ruling. But the key to longevity is fairness and openness, so sometimes sacrifice is needed to boost the spirit of the group. I believe that is why our group has stayed together this long – everyone has been treated fairly. Groups break up when one person decides to be the dictator of the group. My goal is to not only do what I think is right and fair for the group but also serve as a role model to others who will undoubtedly find themselves in similar positions where their wills are against the grain of the group.

Adapting to Changing Legislation

Especially in private practice, it is crucial to be aware of changing legislation. In larger healthcare systems, other departments and administrators, and hospital lawyers may follow legal changes that could affect the practice. In a private practice, the group must all be aware of the changing legal environment to adapt to changes and anticipate them as well.

There are law firms that specialize in medicolegal law. Orthopedic and specialty societies have bulletins that contain information about relevant new legislation. The law can differ by state, so it is helpful to be on the mailing lists of at least one of these firms to be aware of new legislation. There is no need to keep a law firm on retainer in a small or medium-sized practice, since they will happily send these bulletins as advertisements for their services.

Healthcare laws can be state or federal. The Stark Law is an example of a federal mandate, which forbids self-referral for medical care of patients with federal healthcare providers. It, for example, prevents referral to family businesses and only allows this ancillary income to be permitted if it is all under the same federal Tax ID number as the referring practice.

States each have their own regulations. Workman's Compensation has different restrictions and loopholes in each state; some states do not allow the physician to have any self-referrals for physical therapy, epidurals, bracing, etc.; while put in place to avoid self-referral, these also can cause unnecessary delays in patient care due to shifting services between practices, which also can cause prolonged delays of patients being out of work. Regardless, it is important to be aware of what can and cannot be performed and reimbursed, and regarding Workman's Compensation what sort of paperwork and follow-up will be required to care for those patients.

Legislation changes have affected our practice in significant ways. We had operated with one operating room in our surgi-center for years, but suddenly when we were no longer eligible for ambulatory surgical reimbursement because surgicenters were required to have two operating rooms, we had to make a decision to expand our current facility or move to a larger facility in order to continue operating in our surgi-center. We also had our own MRI machine and technician that was both convenient and profitable. When the state of New Jersey enacted legislation that would charge our practice a 2.5% fee on the gross revenue of our entire practice since we had an MRI machine (rather than just a fee on MRI revenue), we had to revisit our cost analysis and deemed that it was no longer financially sustainable to own our own MRI; so we made the decision to sell it. These are just a few examples of how changing legislation brings about real changes to our practice, and how early response to such changes can help maximize operational and financial sustainability for the group.

Managing Expenses

The traditional model of managing a private practice focused on maximizing revenue while providing excellent patient care. However, the past decade has seen downward pressure on revenue due to falling reimbursements as well as increases in fixed costs such as malpractice and employee health insurance. As a result, there has been a move toward managing a lean practice, which focuses on efficient cost management. Before reducing costs on a practice, it is important to understand where they are coming from. These are often classified into direct or indirect costs. Direct costs refer to those that can be traced back to a particular service, product, or practice activity, e.g., staff salaries or office supplies. Conversely, indirect costs refer to those that cannot be traced to a particular product or activity such as rent, utilities, or insurance. Costs can also be evaluated in terms of how they change in response to increasing level of activity, commonly referred to as cost behavior. Fixed costs are those that remain constant over a time period regardless of the level of activity. These include malpractice, health insurance, and rent. Variable costs are those that vary as the volume changes, e.g., patient supplies.

In my practice, the most profound increase in cost that has eroded into net profits has come from fixed costs. This includes malpractice insurance but most notably the costs of health insurance for over 60 employees. Direct costs such as salaries have also increased over this time period. Increases in fixed costs can be mitigated through negotiation of contracts such as signing long-term rent leases for an overall lower annual cost. I would also encourage negotiations with malpractice insurance and employee health insurance providers whenever possible to secure the lowest rates. Legislative pressures have additionally added to fixed costs such as implementation of electronic medical records.

The first area to evaluate when attempting to reduce overall expenses is direct costs, specifically personnel costs which can account for up to 25–30% of a practice's expenses. It is essential to constantly evaluate the necessary number of staff to support each physician in your practice. When possible, reductions in direct cost should be made; however, these must be balanced against ensuring that the physician can focus on generating revenue through patient care. If support staff is cut too low, this can result in the physician performing tasks such as surgical booking, which can be more effectively delegated to staff. Additionally, it is important to look at the roles that each support staff serves to see if those duties can be consolidated. Take stock of the individual skill sets that each staff member possesses to avoid placing an overqualified employee with a higher salary in a job that can be performed by a lower salaried employee.

Maximizing physician–patient interaction is another approach to managing overall revenue streams. In my practice, this entails use of scribes for documentation. Additionally, staff will submit all billing codes after review by the physicians. Notes are printed and placed on the door prior to the patient interaction to minimize the amount of time spent through physician chart review.

Facing Challenges Ahead

Challenges to private practices continue to persist and even evolve in this changing healthcare landscape. Perhaps the greatest challenge will be the emergence of large hospital systems, which have the potential to dominate local marketplaces. These hospital systems have the ability to form exclusive contracts with local or national employers, which can box out small private practices. Additionally, some hospitals are experimenting with their own insurance plans which lock patients into care at their facilities alone. Through aggressive acquisition tactics, hospitals are buying local practices in order to dominate the market. In such situations, private practitioners can combat this by forming "super-groups" which give them access to a larger patient base and more favorable negotiating terms with insurance companies.

Another looming challenge to private practitioners is the ever-increasing role of insurance companies dictating medical care. Not only is there pressure on reimbursements, but insurance companies are beginning to deny routine surgery as unindicted or experimental despite strong scientific evidence to support its efficacy. The time and burden required to conduct peer-to-peer and pre-authorization is unsustainable and costly. A greater role for our professional societies to lobby Congress is required in order to place care back into the surgeon's hands. Changing federal legislation also poses challenges for private practices due to flux in regulation and rules. Currently, practices have been required to invest significant time and money into MACRA despite uncertainty of the future healthcare landscape.

Despite all these challenges, healthy opportunity persists for private practices moving forward. It is likely there will always be a role for private practices as drivers of efficient and outcome-oriented care to the community. The key to success will lie in the ability to constantly adapt to the changing medical landscape while focusing on providing quality patient care.

Recommended Reading

1. Baum N, Bonds RG, Crawford T, Kreder KJ, Shaw K, Stringer T. The complete business guide for a successful medical practice. Cham: Springer; 2015.
2. George B. True north: discover your authentic leadership. San Francisco: Jossey-Bass; 2007.
3. Porter M, Kaplan R, Kahneman D. HBR's 10 must reads 2018: the definitive management ideas of the year from Harvard Business Review. Boston: Harvard Business Review; 2017.

Chapter 7
Leading a Privademic Medical Center: Experience Running the Rothman Institute

Hamadi A. Murphy, Arjun J. Sebastian, Weilong J. Shi, Christie Stawicki, Gregory D. Schroeder, Mike West, and Alexander R. Vaccaro

A Brief History of the Rothman Institute

The Rothman Institute was established in 1970 by Dr. Richard H. Rothman, who at the time, was an orthopedic surgeon and Professor at the University of Pennsylvania. The private practice staff initially only consisted of two surgeons, a nurse, an administrative assistant, and a research coordinator. In 1984, a philanthropist, Walter Annenberg, was very pleased with his treatment and donated $2 million to the practice, allowing the practice to grow and expand. In 1986, Dr. Rothman left Pennsylvania Hospital to accept the Chairman of Orthopedics position at Thomas Jefferson University. In a unique deal, Dr. Rothman was able to bring all the Rothman Institute physicians with him to the university, but still keep the staff of the Rothman Institute privately employed.

Being able to maintain the infrastructure of a private practice allowed the Rothman Institute to respond to changes in healthcare in the 1990s as both private and public insurance payers shifted to a managed care system with the formation of health maintenance organizations (HMOs). These HMOs were successful in limiting costs often at the expense of physician reimbursement rates severely crippling independent or small orthopedic practices. Given these healthcare reforms, and a deliberate strategy to develop community-based offices and strategic health system alliances, the senior partners at the Rothman Institute decided that aggressive expansion while maintaining an academic culture was necessary to survive.

H. A. Murphy (✉) · A. J. Sebastian · W. J. Shi · C. Stawicki · G. D. Schroeder
M. West · A. R. Vaccaro
The Rothman Institute at Thomas Jefferson University, Department of Orthopaedic Surgery, Philadelphia, PA, USA
e-mail: murphypp@mail.uc.edu; Jeff.shi@rothmaninstitute.com; christie.ctawicki@rothmaninstitute.com; greg.schroeder@rothmaninstitute.com; mike.west@rothmaninstitute.com; alex.vaccaro@rothmaninstitute.com

E. C. Makhni et al. (eds.), *Orthopedic Practice Management*,
https://doi.org/10.1007/978-3-319-96938-1_7

The Rothman Institute was able to expand in the Philadelphia, PA, and Southern New Jersey area during a time when many private orthopedic practices were struggling to stay afloat.

The Rothman Institute continued to grow in the decades to come. Today the Rothman Institute employs over 210 physicians and physician assistants. A large part of the reason for the Rothman Institute's success was the ability to thrive in an environment hostile to independent orthopedic offices. Our unique organizational model that combines the benefits of academics and private practice was in large part a reason for this success.

What Is Privademics and Why Privademics Is Desirable?

Dr. Rothman feels that the privademic model employed at the Rothman Institute is a perfect hybrid of different practice philosophies. This model allows the practice the freedom to expand and change as necessary while still maintaining a strong academic core that allows physicians to teach and train future orthopedic surgeons.

Privademic practices allow physicians to determine the quality and method of healthcare delivery without the bureaucratic restrictions of being a large academic institution. By having a balance, physicians can continue to stay up to date and perform clinical and basic science research while still having control of their practice. In fact, a privademic model allows practices to produce as much quality research as large academic centers. The *Journal of Arthroplasty* recently reported the Rothman Institute, a privademic practice, had the most articles accepted in the top orthopedic journals between 2010 and 2014 [1]. In addition, Schoenfield et al. found that the Rothman spine department is the most academically productive spine fellowship program in the country for spine research [2].

Recently, more new physicians have been choosing to join hospitals rather than go into private practice. In addition, many private practices have chosen to shift to the hospital employment model due to the changes in healthcare and limited capital to grow and meet the significant technology (EMR and analytics) requirements to maintain relevancy in the future. The percentage of physician ownership in medical practices went from 57% in 2000 to around 36% in 2013 [3]. While the number of hospital-employed physicians increased by 32% from 2000 to 2011 [4], the number of physicians in a solo practice went down by 17.6% [3].

The evolution of healthcare reform, declining reimbursement, increasing administrative burden, high malpractice costs, and educational debt are all contributors to the shift towards hospital employment [4]. As new physicians struggle with the amount of debt from medical school, this burden tends to direct them to employment opportunities that have less financial risk. In addition, the start-up costs of a new practice can be staggering with the implementation of electronic medical record (EMR) systems costing an estimated $162,047 for a five-physician practice [4]. Furthermore, additional annual total maintenance costs can be as high as $233,297 [4]. Meanwhile, large physician groups or hospitals are able to achieve more affordable bulk pricing for EMR and maintenance per physician [4].

While hospitals and academic centers may seem like a more stable income opportunity, privademic models can match or surpass these centers as well as provide other benefits. Compensation structures offered by privademic practices are very flexible and open to negotiation with individual physicians. Unlike some hospital centers, pay cuts following the first enticing contract are not common. Privademic practices allow physicians to have potential ownership in the practice, where physicians can gain supplementary sources of revenue from ownership stakes in real estate offices, surgery centers, hospitals, along with ancillary services such as diagnostic imaging and physical therapy practices. It provides more opportunity for entrepreneurial and innovative initiatives that are limited to the hospital employment model. However, along with this comes the financial risk associated with any private business, but we believe this further incentivizes physicians to succeed. In an academic or hospital setting, these additional sources of income are absorbed into the hospital budget rather than split among the providers. Lastly, privademic practices also allow physicians to maintain ownership of royalties, intellectual property, and consulting fees.

Another benefit of the privademic model is the organization is free to partner with multiple healthcare organizations allowing for a wide referral range. In addition, strategically joining large healthcare players in various regions helps the practice stay competitive in multiple regions. Having strong relationships with healthcare system partners has been one of the keys to Rothman's success. Mutually beneficial goals and objectives are established with each partner and constant communication has allowed Rothman to grow and succeed in a number of markets. This model also allows for partnering with various entities for ownership stake in ambulatory surgical centers, helping to keep costs low. Only the complex cases need to be referred to large academic hospitals that have higher overhead costs. In addition, despite being the orthopedic program of a large academic center, there is no obligation to share profits with the lower revenue practices of the academic center. Due to the connection to hospital networks and a large academic center, the practice is also able to resist acquisition by other hospital networks while continuing to essentially function as a private practice.

One of the greatest benefits of a privademic model is the fluidity of change. New protocols, processes, and procedures can be implemented in a fast and efficient manner without the bureaucratic process of academic and hospital systems. For example, if a new evidence-based surgical technique is developed, it might take years before an academic center could implement it into practice. However, with a privademic practice, the procedure would be discussed, and if it was thought to be superior, it could be implemented immediately. Physicians are better able to address the needs of their patients and change anything from surgical technique to streamlining a patient experience.

However, there is a downside to the privademic model. While the model does include benefits from academia and the corporate world, there is the added pressure to publish on top of trying to build a new practice. However, while there is more pressure to publish than in a strictly private practice model, the pressure may be less when compared to a pure academic center.

The privademic practice model may be the key to success moving forward in a rapidly changing healthcare environment. In addition to the Rothman Institute, there have been successes in other places with this model. Midwest Orthopaedics at Rush University Medical Center and OrthoCarolina in Charlotte, NC are both highly regarded and nationally recognized programs that have had success with the privademic model.

The Rothman Institute Road to Success

One of the major benefits of running a privademic institution that has allowed the Rothman Institute to flourish is the ability for the physicians to have more autonomy over their practice and more control of the practices business dealings. As a result of The Rothman Institutes unique arrangement with Thomas Jefferson University Hospital, the group has been able to establish and maintain lucrative relationships with other companies in the healthcare industry. This allowed the Rothman Institute to maintain favorable reimbursement rates and margins in the uncertain environment of the 1990s when HMOs were becoming more popular.

Given the institute's success at maneuvering in a changing healthcare landscape, several senior partners in the group helped to found Specialty Care Network Inc. (SCN). SCN was founded as a physician practice management company that focused on assisting practices in the musculoskeletal care arena. SCN saw a great amount of success in its early years resulting in an initial public offering with a market value of over $150 million. The company did well for 3 years after its IPO until some investors pulled out due to a failed merger. The failed merger of two large physician practice management (PPM) organizations (Phycare and Medpartners) disrupted the entire PPM market. Many of the institutional investors left the sector and stock prices plummeted to a low point; reorganization and/or bankruptcy crippled the entire PPM market. After the Rothman Institute's exit from SCN, the senior partners developed a new strategic plan for the growth and development of the practice.

The senior shareholders agreed that they wanted to maintain the academic and teaching culture of the Institute and developed a strategy to establish multiple satellite offices in surrounding communities to grow the practice. Throughout the growth of the organization, Rothman has maintained a very disciplined and conservative financial philosophy. Early on, the shareholders adopted a "no debt" policy. As growth occurred the shareholders would fund all expansions, investments, and capital expenditures through the use of retained earnings. This still holds true as of 2017. The growth strategy of the Rothman Institute would be based off of the Hub & Spoke concept that many privademic institutions today have been founded on (Fig. 7.1).

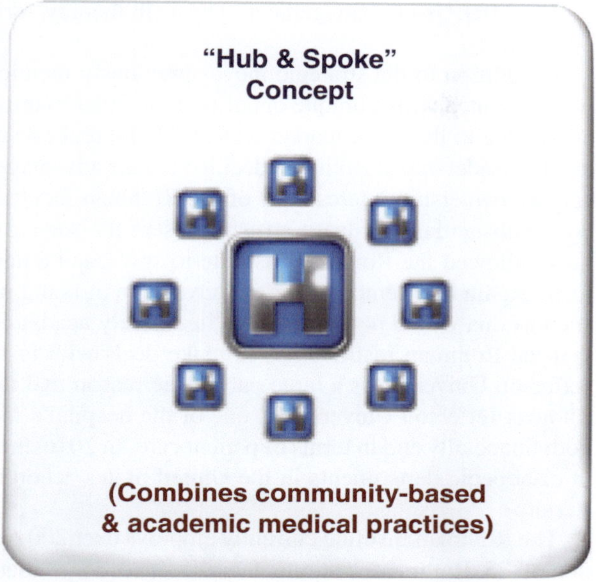

Fig. 7.1 Graphic representation of Hub & Spoke model with a large academic center serving as the hub

Given the Rothman Institute's relationship with Thomas Jefferson University Hospital, their main hospital campus in center city Philadelphia would serve as the "Hub," and the multiple community Rothman Institute locations in South Jersey and the Philadelphia metro area would serve as the so-called spokes. The advantages of the Rothman community office locations are twofold. First, they allow for greater convenience to patients living near those offices, and second, these facilities have lower operating costs, which allows the Rothman Institute to improve on profit margins. The Hub & Spoke model of the Rothman Institute also includes several ambulatory surgery centers in the Philadelphia and South Jersey area as well as a specialty orthopedic hospital in Bensalem, PA.

The specialty hospital in Bensalem, PA was purchased as a joint venture with multiple healthcare systems including Nueterra healthcare, Thomas Jefferson University, and Holy Redeemer Health System. This facility includes 60,000 sq feet of medical office space and 60,000 sq feet of operating facilities with a total of 6 operating rooms and 24 patient beds. This specialty hospital, which was branded as the Rothman Orthopaedic Specialty Hospital (ROSH), is another example of how Rothman has positioned itself for success with its strategic plan. ROSH has been one of the most successful endeavors that the Rothman Institute has undertaken, and has been recognized as the highest-ranking hospital in the United States for Medicare value-based purchasing in 2016. Between 2009 and 2014, Rothman continued its investment in ASCs establishing relationships with multiple facilities in the Delaware Valley region. In the same span of time, Rothman has expanded from 10 to 20 community offices in South Jersey and Philadelphia area. Many of the Rothman community locations offer ancillary and non-operative services including

X-ray, MRI, pain management, physical therapy, orthotics, hand therapy, and nutrition.

In addition to the strategic moves previously mentioned, the Rothman Institute was presented with a unique opportunity in 2009 to improve upon its financial situation. Due to the stock market crash of 2008, real estate prices were at a low point and the leadership at Rothman decided to take advantage. The decision was made to acquire ownership interest in 9 of the Rothman facilities; this decreased our lease costs substantially as lease costs represent the second highest practice cost. This move allowed the Rothman Institute to save capital and invest more in other ventures. Again this demonstrates the advantage of being privademic as an acquisition such as this would not be possible in a purely academic department. The freedom that the Rothman Institute has to make deals with institutions outside of Thomas Jefferson University is a large part of the reason that the orthopedic department at Thomas Jefferson University is one of the hospital's most successful departments, both financially and in terms of patient care. In 2016, the department was ranked 7th in orthopedic departments in the United States according to US News and World Report.

The Rothman Institute currently employs over 200 physicians and PA's operating out of 23 Rothman Institute facilities and 35 affiliated hospitals. In 2016, the Rothman Institute had over 780,000 patient visits and performed 50,788 surgeries. It is no question that our unique arrangement with Jefferson University Hospitals has allowed the Rothman Institute to see increased success in recent years. Rothman has benefitted from having the support and backing that comes with being affiliated with an academic institution and Rothman has also benefitted from having the ability to independently make business decisions that are best for the physician practice free of bureaucratic hassles.

In 2014, Dr. Alexander R. Vaccaro was appointed as the President and Chairman of the Rothman Institute. Since taking over, Dr. Vaccaro has been a champion of the Rothman Institute's growth strategy and is working to expand the practice into North Jersey and New York City. Given recent shifts in the healthcare landscape that include increasing physician employment, increasing scrutiny of high-cost procedures, and declining reimbursement, both Dr. Rothman and Dr. Vaccaro see opportunities for continued expansion into becoming a fully integrated medical home for the duration of musculoskeletal care.

During Dr. Vaccaro's tenure at Rothman, he has worked to make the organization more transparent. He has been very open with the communication of relevant data and has been very engaging with the physicians so that they feel more a part and have more input in the decision making. He has also been very adamant about dealing with unacceptable physician behavior and deals directly with the issues, being completely fair regarding how he handles things. He has also accelerated the strategic initiatives and holds everyone at the company accountable, including himself.

Dr. Vaccaro himself sets the standards when it comes to work ethic in both clinical and academic/teaching disciplines. He has reorganized the physician leadership through the Board of Council, which has allowed feedback and input from physicians related to operational issues. This was updated from our historic manner of dealing with or not dealing with issues, which has been by service line. Now at The Rothman Institute, monthly meetings are held, and the Board of Council representatives (physicians) meet with the senior management team to address operational or regional issues.

Conclusion

In conclusion, physicians entering the workforce today face many complex decisions regarding choosing the ideal practice model that fits their short- and long-term career goals. Privademics is a practice model that offers physicians the advantage of having the resources of an academic center while having the ability to independently maintain control of the business aspects of the practice. This is a model that has allowed the Rothman Institute to thrive in the 1990s, early 2000s, and into the current time. Because of this unique practice structure, the Rothman Institute is a leader in the field of orthopedics and is now poised to continue its expansion into nearby area markets and beyond.

References

1. Formby P, Pavey G, Van Blarcum G, Mack A, Newman M. An analysis of research from Faculty at U.S. Adult reconstruction fellowships. J Arthoplast. 2015;30:2376–9.
2. Schoenfeld AJ, Bhalla A, George J, Harris MB, Bono CM. Academic productivity and contributions to the literature among spine surgery fellowship faculty. Spine J. 2015;15(10):2126–31.
3. Satiani B, Vaccaro P. A critical appraisal of physician-hospital integration models. J Vasc Surg. 2010;51(4):1046–53.
4. Charles AG, Ortiz-Pujols S, Ricketts T, Fraher E, Neuwahl S, Cairns B, et al. The employed surgeon: a changing professional paradigm. JAMA Surg. 2013;148(4):323.

Chapter 8
Recruitment and Department Expansion

William N. Levine

Departmental Assessment

The critical first steps necessary for an incoming chairman include assessment of the current faculty, departmental milestones and metrics, and the opportunities for growth and expansion. This process should be done at the macro- (30,000-foot view) and micro levels. From the macro level, how many surgeons are currently employed and working in the department? How many surgeons are in each subspecialty and are they all working to maximum capacity? These questions will help to inform decision-making as a business plan and mission/vision statement begin to be formulated.

As a former member of the department for which I was named Chairman, I had a distinct advantage over an external recruit since I was well aware of the areas of opportunity for faculty recruitment and departmental expansion. We had a relatively small faculty when I was named Chairman due to faculty retirements and several relocations of former faculty who had moved before the announcement.

One of the key elements to our strategy was to employ the Advisory Board to help provide market analysis, local and regional benchmarks, and an overview of the competitive landscape. This data ultimately provided incredibly powerful information for us to make the case to the hospital leadership where, when, and how many faculty recruits were appropriate to consider based on patient-centered needs. The Advisory Board is a best practice firm that combines market research, technology and consulting to improve the performance of healthcare organizations. Data-driven recruitment allowed a proactive approach rather than a reactive one and the hospital leadership responded favorably to this.

W. N. Levine
New York Presbyterian/Columbia University Medical Center, Department of Orthopedic Surgery, New York, NY, USA
e-mail: wnl1@columbia.edu

E. C. Makhni et al. (eds.), *Orthopedic Practice Management*,
https://doi.org/10.1007/978-3-319-96938-1_8

Philosophy of Recruitment/Departmental Expansion

Alignment of vision and mission and transparent communication are critical to every chairperson's ultimate success or failure in their role as the leader of the department. Every time a decision to recruit a specific subspecialty faculty member was initiated, I would meet with the current faculty in that subspecialty to discuss with them the recruitment process, whom we had identified as potential recruits, and to solicit names from our faculty of desirable candidates. The subspecialty Chief/Director has to be 100% supportive of same-specialty recruitments or the process will fail miserably. In addition, buy-in from the other subspecialty faculty is integral to successful recruitment as an uninformed or unwilling faculty member can and will likely poison the well – either knowingly or unknowingly. Once the decision to bring in a faculty recruit has been made, we go to great lengths to provide a professional, meaningful, and efficient recruitment process.

The Recruitment Process

"New Versus Seasoned?"

The decision to recruit a fresh out of fellowship surgeon compared to a seasoned veteran depends on several factors – subspecialty division size, hospital resources, and hospital type/operating room availability.

Subspecialty Division Size

The first question that needs to be addressed is, "Do we need another surgeon for this subspecialty?" Market analysis, hospital location, and surgeon-specific metrics can help answer this question. Key practice metrics include new patient-surgery conversion ratio, wait time for new patients, new patient/follow-up patient office visit fill rate, and operating room fill rate. Our practice dashboard provided to every surgeon each month includes these key indicators as well as others. We aim for a new patient/surgical conversion ratio of 4:1 or lower – meaning that for every 4 patients seen by the surgeon at least 1 patient is scheduled for surgery. If this ratio is higher than 4:1, then we implement strategies to address this – hiring of nonoperative providers and fine-tuning front-end screening with our appointment scheduling team. Wait time for new patient office visits is a key practice indicator that the University's Faculty Practice Organization (FPO) sets at 9 days maximum. Our department policy, however, is that any patient who calls for a new appointment will be accommodated that day if they wish – we achieve this metric by offering every new patient the opportunity to be seen by a provider that day whether it be a nurse practitioner, nonoperative musculoskeletal physician, or a surgeon from that specific subspecialty if the one which they specifically asked for is unavailable.

New patient/follow-up patient outpatient clinic fill rate is provided to each faculty member by location so that we can easily assess the needs for another provider in that area. Finally, operative fill rate is the critical metric to determine the need for additional recruitment and the area that makes most people nervous about recruiting another surgeon in their subspecialty. My own observation is that young surgeons are inherently wary of bringing on new surgeons if they are still feeling their practice is not mature.

Hospital Resources

Sharing the vision with the hospital leadership dictates whether the recruit will be fresh out of fellowship or someone whose practice you hope to transfer (if they are currently at another system in your area). The financial implications are obvious – younger surgeons cost less than the established surgeons. However, the financial risk may be greater given that the cost to the organization may not be recovered if the surgeon does not successfully develop a sustainable practice beyond the initial guaranteed contract time (3 years in our system). On the other hand, an established surgeon with a strong following and track record of success may hit the ground running and the return on investment may be felt much quicker. Care here to not overpay the established surgeon is critical to avoid "sweetheart" deals is critically important as I have personally seen these arrangements backfire around the country.

Hospital Type/Operating Room Availability

As mentioned above, the paradigm has clearly shifted within the past several years with the advent of large hospital systems buying smaller hospitals, private practice groups, and clinics. Operating room availability is the most prized resource necessary for any recruitment. Having mentored hundreds of residents and fellows over the years, it never ceases to amaze the number of times someone is recruited without guaranteed operating room time. While not an absolute fatal flaw it is concerning to me when this feature is not guaranteed since the ultimate success of the recruit will be tied directly to their clinical productivity. In addition, the hospital type is important for consideration – do the hospital and community support a recruit with this specific skill set? Are there resources necessary for subspecialty trained surgeons or would that person be better off at the main hospital where those resources already exist? Typically, hospital systems do now want to have to duplicate all the extensive resources at each hospital but instead create an environment where the "bread and butter" cases can be performed readily at the affiliated hospitals but that if the patient requires more specialized equipment, expertise, they will be referred to the main hospital.

After evaluating all these issues, we decide if we want to hire a new surgeon versus recruiting one with more experience (either local or national). We then develop a business plan which must be approved by the hospital and medical school providing us with the green light to proceed with the recruitment process.

Initial Contact

Initial contact is made with the potential faculty member and a telephone meeting is coordinated to gauge interest, share the vision, and determine if bringing them in for a formal recruitment visit is mutually agreeable. I place a great deal of importance in this initial communication to avoid unnecessary recruitment visits which delay the process, increase costs, and lead to potential recruitment burnout for the faculty. For example, if the potential recruit is not from your geographic area and they have family elsewhere it may just not be the right fit. Even more important is to understand early in the process whether the recruit's significant other, partner, or spouse would be willing to move to your area. Far too many recruitment anecdotes exist where multiple visits were had only to have the recruit end the process by saying, "my spouse decided that he/she could not move to this area." I strive to make this a never event in the recruitment process as best as possible.

First Visit

The first recruitment visit is designed for the faculty recruit to formally meet with the Chairman, Program Director, subspecialty colleagues, several other faculty members including senior and more junior recruits, our Departmental Administrator, and Chief Financial Officer, and depending on the recruit, hospital and or medical school leadership. A social gathering either the night before the interview day or the night of the interview day is typically arranged depending on the recruit's timeline to return home. This visit is designed to assess "fit" of the recruit. Camaraderie, culture, and collegiality are the key features for the success of the group. The group dynamic can be destroyed if a new person coming in does not have the shared values, vision and mission of the organization.

Faculty/Staff/Other Assessment

After the first visit, feedback is solicited from everyone who interacted with the recruit including those who formally interviewed and anyone else who came into contact with the recruit during the visit. In addition, feedback from the administrative staff assigned to the faculty recruit's visit for the day is important since the day is a long one and our administrative staff have decades of experience and often provide a great litmus test as to the recruit's personality, patience, and empathetic qualities.

Second Visit

Depending on the success or failure of the first visit, we will often proceed with a second more comprehensive visit. Here, the recruit will have the opportunity to learn more about the finances of the organization, the compensation plan, and the "nitty-gritty" about becoming a member of the department. We will invite the spouse or significant other to this visit if they did not come to the first visit. Buy-in from the spouse/significant other (as highlighted above) is ultimately as important; or more important; than virtually every other factor. If the recruit has research interests, we will coordinate dedicated time with our research team during the second visit to assess needs, space, and resources.

Formal Offer

After going through the recruitment process, we will make a determination of the fit and viability of the specific applicant. If the faculty and administration all feel it is a go, then the business plan will be converted into a formal offer letter which will be sent to the recruit. The offer letter outlines the terms of agreement including the time (typically 3 years for a new recruit or 3–4 years for a veteran recruit), financial agreement, productivity bonus discussion, and general hospital and medical school policy/guidelines.

Faculty Hiring: Keys to Success

Once the faculty member has been successfully recruited and signed their offer letter a number of wheels are set in motion. First, the credentialing process has to begin immediately – this can take 3–6 months depending on the organization and is not something that you should take for granted will happen immediately. The recruit needs to be hyper-vigilant to ensure that all paperwork is submitted in a timely manner and that there are no missing data as this will serve to delay the process. (I am aware of many situations where start times were delayed by as much as 6 months due to failure to promptly get all materials submitted). Determination of the recruit's weekly schedule is often analogous to playing with a Rubik's cube – move one color on one side and the opposite side's color is moved in an unintended and disruptive way! Selecting key office sites (again viewing it from where the needs are in the organization), ambulatory surgicenter time (if appropriate for the specific subspecialty), and operating room time are the critical components to the successful transition into the department.

Mentorship

Mentorship for young faculty is critical to their success. Hiring someone and then letting them fly by the seat of their pants should hopefully be viewed as an anachronistic practice from days gone by. Assignment of a faculty mentor can be an effective mechanism to ensure that the new faculty member feels supported in their new job. The Division chief may or may not be the best person for this job so it needs to be assessed individually. Frequent meetings with the Chairman or supervisory partner is helpful to ensure that the transition is going smoothly. Creation of a culture of support and assistance is the ultimate goal. The typical academic paradigm has looked something like this: take the youngest, most inexperienced surgeon, give them end of day operating room time, provide insufficient support (PG-2 resident), and top it off with the most complex cases. In short, nobody would ever design a system like that but in fact, it is not uncommon to see this around the country. Therefore, creating a culture where faculty support and help each other and where it is expected that asking for help is the norm, not the exception. Scheduling cases with a senior partner is mandatory in some practices but certainly something that should be encouraged with new faculty to help ease the transition from fellow to faculty.

Summary

Faculty recruitment and departmental expansion are critically important components for all chairpersons in the country. The lifeline of the department is having a vibrant, robust clinical machine with surgeons and physicians who efficiently and safely take care of patients. Identifying faculty members who share the goals and objectives of the departmental leadership is integral to the success of the department. For potential faculty members, understanding the specific nature of the position including hospital location, type of practice (academic vs. privademic vs. private practice), and the reasons for the recruitment will help steer you into the best fit possible.

Recommended Reading

1. McChrystal S, Collins T. Team of teams: new rules of engagement for a complex world; 2015.
2. McKeown G. Essentialism: the disciplined pursuit of less. New York: Crown Business; 2014.

Chapter 9
Implementing Outcomes Collection in Clinical Practice

Fabien Meta, Vincent A. Lizzio, and Eric C. Makhni

Importance and Relevance of Collecting Outcomes Data

Anecdotally, many clinicians will concur that a patient expresses infinite gratitude when function has been restored and pain has been relieved. However, the patient as an individual may have a skewed perspective of the relative value provided by a given treatment, as there are limited avenues of comparison readily accessible to the patient. To put this in perspective, a rotator cuff repair patient may be disappointed because their next-door neighbor's rotator cuff repair has succeeded in allowing the neighbor to return to gardening without pain and impairment, but this patient still has difficulty with simple tasks such as reaching for the top shelf in the cupboard. This disappointment could stem from an unequal comparison, for they may be at different timepoints in rehabilitation progression. They might also have had different severities of rotator cuff tears. It might also be plausible that level of function was unequal to begin with based on age, body habitus, strength level, and pre-injury ability. It is the provider's responsibility to adjust the patient's expectations, not an easy task unless tangible data about their disease trajectory can be presented and tracked. This brief example illustrates why any orthopedic surgeon should be interested in collecting data on patient outcomes. They are not solely reserved for the academically ambitious.

More globally, patient outcomes play a vital role in quantifying value in medicine and orthopedics. Patients and healthcare policy makers alike are interested in

F. Meta · V. A. Lizzio
Wayne State University School of Medicine, Henry Ford Hospital, Department of Orthopedic Surgery, Detroit, MI, USA
e-mail: fmeta@med.wayne.edu; vlizzio@med.wayne.edu

E. C. Makhni (✉)
Division of Sports Medicine, Department of Orthopedic Surgery, Henry Ford Health System, West Bloomfield, MI, USA

E. C. Makhni et al. (eds.), *Orthopedic Practice Management*,
https://doi.org/10.1007/978-3-319-96938-1_9

determining whether a chosen intervention can provide improvement at a reasonable cost. As a general economic principle, value can be viewed as a relationship of quality per related cost. Numerically, this can be represented as an equation of quality as the numerator and cost as the denominator. Outcomes then become the measure of quality, while the denominator (cost) can be readily determined [1]. This outlines the transition from volume to value-based reimbursement. For a procedural profession, such as orthopedic surgery, this is paramount.

Outcomes are becoming the fulcrum of leveraging payment as a physician, but it did not start this way. Originally, diligent outcomes collection was seen as a solution to the shocking reports of the frequency of medical mistakes by the Institute of Medicine (IOM) at the turn of the century [2, 3]. This gave birth to accountability in healthcare. As a result, we are now seeing models for accountability in orthopedics with programs such as Comprehensive Care for Joint Replacement (CJR). This initiative includes several health systems and hospitals across the country, and holds hospitals accountable for quality and cost of an episode of care related to major joint replacement for Medicare beneficiaries [4].

Evidently, this reality places an urgency on implementing an outcomes collection system in the majority of orthopedic practices. In an ideal setting, outcomes should be consistently collected whether the focus is academic research or quality of clinical care. However, successful implementation of an outcomes collection system relies heavily on optimization of workflow in the clinic, all the while being mindful of the Health Insurance and Portability and Accountability Act (HIPAA) as most existing electronic health records do not have provisions to efficiently capture and store this once considered extraneous health information. This chapter will attempt to construct the ground-level details required for effective and efficient outcomes collection in most practice models.

Objective Outcomes

Traditionally, objective outcomes are the most commonly collected outcomes in clinical practice. In orthopedics, the most relevant objective outcomes include strength, range of motion, imaging, intraoperative findings, and adverse events, among others. In the following section, we describe how each of these outcomes can be reliably and efficiently collected in an orthopedic practice.

Strength

Assessing strength is a staple of the physical exam and one of the most commonly reported outcomes in orthopedic surgery. Muscular weakness can be caused by either structural defects or excessive pain. Nearly all activities of daily living rely on adequate strength; thus, its impact on lifestyle cannot be understated.

There are several methods of collecting strength data on patients while in the clinic, the most common of which is an assessment on a 5-point grading scale. In this model, Grade 0 represents no contraction or muscle movement and Grade 5 represents normal muscular strength, with the other grades defined by the ability to move against resistance and gravity. Many providers will often include a "+" or "–" in order to add further distinction within each grade. This assessment is routinely performed during the physical exam due to its simplicity and convenience. However, while this evaluation is easy to perform in the clinical setting, it has limited utility as a research tool because of the qualitative nature of the exam and the wide variation of weakness that qualifies for each grade.

In contrast, handheld dynamometers can be used to quantify muscle strength. These portable instruments can be easily used in the clinic and measure the isometric force exerted by a muscle [5]. During the assessment, the provider holds the dynamometer against the patient's limb and asks the patient to push against the instrument with their full effort. While slightly more cumbersome than the subjective assessment, this method is much more specific and reliable for tracking progress in recovery. Unfortunately, this instrument can only measure strength in an isometric manner, and is unable to measure dynamic strength.

The "gold standard" for measuring strength is often done by isokinetic dynamometers, such as the Biodex (USA). These instruments will measure maximum strength across the full range of motion in a single plane across an isolated joint, and can more comprehensively and accurately assess dynamic strength. These devices are expensive, take up a large amount of space, and are generally not practical for routine clinical use.

Range of Motion

Like strength, the range of motion of an affected limb has a large impact on quality of life. For this reason, assessing both active and passive range of motion is a standard part of the routine clinical exam. Traditionally, clinicians have used visually estimated range of motion or reported the ability of their patient to reach common musculoskeletal landmarks. For example, the internal rotation of the glenohumeral joint is often reported as the most cephalad vertebra that the patient can reach (e.g., L1, L2, etc.). These estimations, although quick and convenient, are not as reliable as when using objective measurement tools [6].

A goniometer is the most reliable instrument for objectively assessing range of motion in the clinic setting. This simple instrument has a single pivot point that anchors two arms, the intersection of which quantifies the angle. After the patient has performed the desired task, the clinician puts the pivot of the goniometer directly over the fulcrum of the joint and aligns the arms along the proximal and distal segments in order to determine the angle. For both clinical and research purposes, the goniometer is the most convenient and practical instrument for accurately assessing range of motion in orthopedic patients.

Imaging

Routine clinical imaging is commonly utilized to compliment a patient's history and physical exam. Although imaging does not always correlate strongly with symptoms or clinical progress [7–9], it still provides important information related to disease process and treatment options. While computed tomography (CT) and magnetic resonance imaging (MRI) require separate appointments with radiology, other imaging modalities – such as radiographs and ultrasonography – can be quickly captured and interpreted in the clinic setting, provided that this equipment is available. Thus, the vast majority of patients seen in clinic will have at least some available imaging for data collection.

While evaluation of radiographs, ultrasound, CT, and MRI largely relies on subjective interpretation, there are a number of well-defined measurements that can be utilized for collecting objective data. These distances and angles can easily be calculated on standard imaging software (e.g., GE PACS). Since images are saved and stored in patient charts, these images can be analyzed retrospectively and data collection can take place outside of clinic hours.

Intraoperative Findings

Although not an outcome collected in the clinic, documenting intraoperative diagnoses and procedures is an essential component for comprehensive evaluation of patient outcomes. This information provides the opportunity to define comparison groups that clinical outcome data can be compared against, both before and after the procedure is performed.

Most pertinent intraoperative findings and procedures should be available in the operative note; however, it is not reasonable to expect every aspect of the case to be described in the detail required for comprehensive data collection. Thus, aside from the information in a standard op note, the surgeon must decide what information to document for prospective or retrospective analysis and record this data in a consistent manner so that it can then be mined and organized into a template spreadsheet for future statistical analysis. Ultimately, it is easier to decide what information to record – and the manner in which to record it – prior to initiating a collection system so that the data can be easily translated into a convenient spreadsheet format, since retrospective data collection may be difficult and inconsistent. It is often most efficient to create a standard data set for each diagnosis and procedure. Important data to collect during surgery may include operation time, blood loss, details involving diagnosis (e.g., describing the status of each individual tendon instead of generally stating "rotator cuff tear"), size and type of implants, specific technique used for procedure, and anything else that may be of interest for future studies.

Adverse Events

It is important to document complications and other adverse events that have occurred since the last clinic visit or identified while in clinic as part of outcome data collection. Adverse events will undoubtedly impact both subjective and objective outcomes. Thus, information that surrounds these events, such as the type of complication, the duration of time since surgery, or admission to the hospital, to name a few, should be recorded in order to provide context for that patient's clinical outcomes.

Subjective Outcomes

Unlike objective outcomes, subjective outcomes are less observer-based, and more focused on the sentiment of the patient. This allows the patient to become a stakeholder in the process of delivering care. Naturally, this perspective has inherent importance, and was one of the six constructs that constitute quality healthcare according to the Institute of Medicine [10]. Classically, subjective outcomes employ the use of patient-reported outcomes (PROs) to gauge general health, pain, function, return to activity and even patient satisfaction. Understanding these principles will guide effective outcomes collection.

Patient-Reported Outcomes

Patient-reported outcomes are typically collected using validated questionnaires and are categorized by anatomic, disease-specific, or general health constructs. The advent of PROs is well-documented and increasingly popular in an era of patient-centered care [11]. Effectively choosing the right PRO measures for your practice requires a systematic approach. First and foremost, the surgeon must decide whether to target an anatomic region, disease, or general health for assessment. In addition, there are several other points of deliberation. These include assessing a PRO for validated scores, appropriate psychometrics, ease of use for the patient, ease of scoring and comprehension for physician, standardized use, and cost considerations [12, 13]. Validity of scores and psychometric properties, such as responsiveness, reliability, internal consistency, floor/ceiling effects, and ability to measure clinically meaningful change, are especially important when considering reporting outcomes for a research purpose, and can be done through investigation of PRO measures in readily available scientific literature [14]. Appropriate assessment of these properties also allows the provider to have confidence that the chosen PRO measure adequately targets the desired clinical question for the patient (Fig. 9.1).

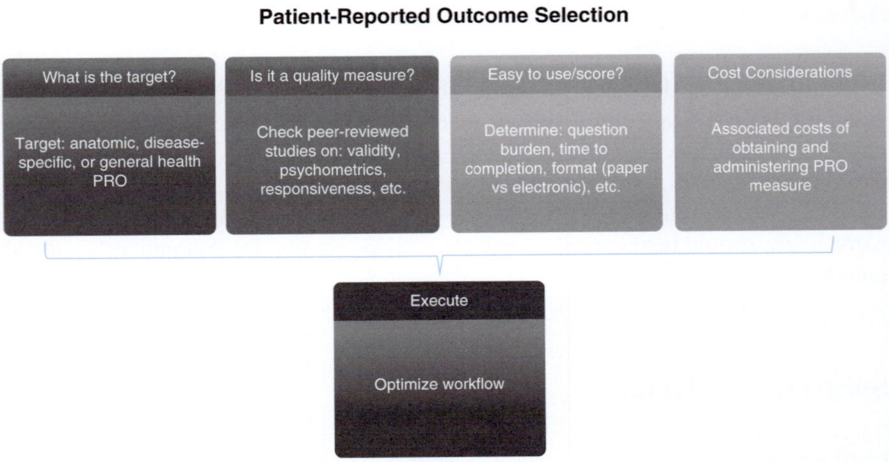

Fig. 9.1 Factors to consider when selecting patient-reported outcomes

Choosing appropriate anatomic/disease-specific PRO measures, and delving into advantages and disadvantages of each, requires a book of its own. The scope of this chapter is to serve as a guide for implementing an outcomes collection system in the ordinary orthopedic practice. Having said that, there are important points to consider when creating a comprehensive outcomes collection system.

Understandably, including a disease-specific or anatomic PRO measure makes sense in terms of assessing your patients' index problem and subsequent trajectory. However, we propose a general health questionnaire, which provides a better perspective of the global impact the injury has on the patient. This sentiment is also shared by the American Academy of Orthopedic Surgeons (AAOS) [13]. Numerous ones have been studied in orthopedic literature. Most commonly used general health questionnaires include the 36 question, short form (SF-36), derived from the medical outcomes study (MOS) and the briefer 12 question version, SF-12. These surveys use 8 subscales to create two composite scores, the mental component summary (MCS) and the physical component summary (PCS) [15, 16]. The MOS SF-36v2 is a commercial system and maintained by Optum, Inc., which allows for easy population norm-based scoring, but with an associated cost. In a busy practice, the 12-question option is likely more attractive, and is shown to correlate well to the 36-question option [17].

There are also cost-effective alternatives such as the RAND-36 (VR-36) which is the original version of the MOS-derived SF-36, and is used in the Veteran's Affairs hospital system, but is available for free from the RAND corp. The questions are virtually the same, but the VR-36 requires manual scoring using the guidelines outlined in the RAND Corporation webpage [18]. Another readily available, cost-effective option, is the EuroQol-5D (EQ-5D), developed by the EuroQol Research Foundation [19]. This is another extensively validated general health measure, and despite its European origin, normative scores are available for the general US population [20]. The strength of this questionnaire originates from its brief nature, 5 questions, plus a visual analog scale question, and the ability to convert scores to health utility states, in order to facilitate health utility research. Costing a nominal license fee for clinical use, or free licensing if used solely for research, the EQ-5D is another strong choice.

Patient-Reported Outcome Measurement Information System (PROMIS)

The variety of PROs developed over decades of research, including general health questionnaires, has created a demand for a standardized PRO system. The National Institutes of Health have recognized this, and has focused funding efforts to develop the Patient-Reported Outcome Measurement Information System (PROMIS). This marks an exciting evolution in outcomes collection as it has a created a centralized location for a rich assortment of validated questionnaires organized into domains of health, such as global health, physical health, mental health, and social health [21]. Another strength of this system stems from its near-universal applicability of its item banks to an array of adult and pediatric populations. However, the measures with the greatest orthopedic relevance within the PROMIS bank of outcome measurements include the PROMIS Physical Function (PF) and PROMIS Pain Interference (PI). These questionnaires allow patients to self-report levels of functional capabilities (PF), and hindrance of day-to-day activities due to pain (PI)—an innovative way to assess pain.

The advantages to the PROMIS initiative include the ability to use static short forms (SF) and dynamic computerized adaptive test (CAT) forms. The CAT forms are an inventive method to reduce the question burden on patients by determining relevant subsequent questions based on the previous response. These questions are chosen from a bank based on item-response theory [22, 23]. The requirement of a computer may be a drawback of the CAT system; however, advancements in handheld/tablet computers have made this less of an obstacle in recent years.

Psychological Outcomes: Are They Valuable to an Orthopedic Practice?

Although consistently under the radar, tracking PROs regarding psychological status before, during, and after recovery represents an untapped assessment that can alter and even help predict patient recovery. For instance, in ACL reconstruction, numerous studies have indicated that psychological factors, such as motivation and self-efficacy, affect outcomes and rehabilitation [24–26]. Even significant relationships have been shown between self-esteem levels and objective findings such as functional test performance, as well as other disease-specific PRO measures [26].

Long-term outcomes can also be affected, as one study demonstrated; depression has an impact on outcomes even as far out as 5 years from knee arthroplasty [27]. The well-apparent role that psychological well-being can have on physical outcomes for patients has been recognized by PROMIS as well. Consequently, several mental health assessments are available in CAT and static formats, such as PROMIS Depression.

Regarding musculoskeletal care, tracking these outcomes may prove especially beneficial in traditionally deemed "difficult" patients. Many times in orthopedics a patient's emotions can be affected by expectations of their outcomes [28]. As a healthcare provider, baseline psychological scores may help frame physician–patient communication, and comparison with postoperative psychological scores may provide an opportunity to appreciate the impact restoration of function may have in a patient's emotional health.

Return to Activity, a Milestone Worth Merit

Related to emotional health is the track to recovery from injury, as it can be a tumultuous journey for many patients, often involving dedication to structured rehabilitation. The culmination of patient adherence and dedication is marked by return to pre-injury level of function, largely considered one of the most important clinical outcomes by patients [29]. This critical achievement in recovery progression can be considered a "milestone," and we propose that all orthopedic providers track the time required to return to this level of function. Such an important statistic is underreported when compared to PRO scores [30], which may have arbitrary importance to the patient. Thus, milestone reporting would allow clinicians to report metrics most important to patients. For example, a collegiate football player likely is not interested in what his six-month IKDC (PRO) score is, but rather when he will be able to return to full participation in sport. Similarly, the laborer is interested in time to return to full work capacity, as this can impact overall treatment costs by affecting earnings and job status. In fact, some estimates approximate that up to 40% of direct and indirect costs of hip and knee arthroplasties are associated outside the acute care phase, with roughly 75% of total estimated costs associated with time off from work [31]. In addition to the evident patient relevance, the significant advantage in reporting time to return to work/sport/activity is the ability to quickly and easily report even in the busiest of practices.

Patient Satisfaction: The Basics

Patient satisfaction can be thought of as a surrogate summary of the overall healthcare experience. High levels of satisfaction have been associated with increased market share, financial gains, decreased malpractice claims, and improved reimbursement rates [32]. As a result, satisfaction has already made its way into compensation formulas, such as ones used by the Centers for Medicare & Medicaid Services (CMS) [32]. Understanding how to capture this critical outcome may prove beneficial for patients and the viability of practices alike.

Important factors that often influence the spectrum of satisfaction include pain relief, functional restoration, fulfilling expectations, cost of treatment, hardship endured during recovery, quality of clinic and staff, and time commitment to the healthcare process. However, these components may not have an equal impact on satisfaction and some authors propose that they can be categorized as role-players within two related, but different, concepts: satisfaction with the outcome of care, and satisfaction with the process of care [33]. One attempts to describe healthcare quality while the other focuses on service quality. Such broad constructs within satisfaction likely drives the variety of measures used, with many of them having uncertain validity [34], and many others not originally designed for satisfaction [35–37]. As a result, there is a lack of consensus in orthopedic literature indicating optimal measures for satisfaction, but for the research-focused practitioner, the validated Patient Satisfaction Questionnaire developed by the AAOS may provide a viable option for use [33]. Other options include surveys focusing on fulfilling expectations for specific surgeries developed by the Hospital for Special Surgery [38, 39], as it is well known that unmet expectations can be a negative predictor of satisfaction [40]. Still, the majority of orthopedic practices may benefit from brief, custom questionnaires focusing on questions such as: "Would you have the surgery/treatment again?" or "How satisfied are you with the function of your injured/surgically fixed area?". These examples can be quantified with the use of a visual analog scale (VAS) ranging from 0 to 100, offering tangible data to traditionally anecdotal questions.

How to Collect Outcomes in Your Practice

Integrating the introductory knowledge regarding the importance, relevance, and variety of patient outcomes with practical application know-how can propel a successful outcomes collection system. This section highlights the largely overlooked logistics for sustaining outcomes collection without interrupting your practice from a financial and/or operations standpoint.

Equipment, Staff, and Clinic Flow

Just as with any endeavor to improve and change a practice, there can be a significant learning curve associated with the trial and error of implementing an outcomes collection system. Expenses will inevitably come in the form of time and money, with the former decreasing as routines are developed, and the latter consistent over time aside from startup costs. While seemingly a significant investment, insurers, payers, and quality monitoring agencies are increasingly valuing data masses to determine high-quality care. Preparation regarding equipment, support staff, and clinic flow before launch can mitigate the growing pains of obtaining this valuable data.

For a comprehensive outcomes system, there are several key pieces of equipment needed. Primarily, for efficiency, data collection should be done electronically with computers and tablets as the principal tools for collection. These measures can reduce data errors and administrative burden, potentially driving costs down in the long run. Computers offer more computing power and familiarity of use by a broader range of patients, but tablets offer versatility, portability, and secure storability. In fact, the use of tablets for collection as well as SMS message reminders have been shown to be an effective solution to get surgical patients to fill out PRO scores at high response rates [41]. Furthermore, the tablets or computers should have wireless network connectivity to ensure that data entered can be directly uploaded to any central repositories. Whether computers or tablets are used, a collection interface or platform is needed as a medium for organized collection and can be considered a virtual piece of equipment. Many popular orthopedic options are mentioned in the next section. In short, commercial systems cost more but essentially run hands-free with automatic solutions to issues such as secure data storage and tech support. Also, extensive libraries allow many established platforms to have readily available questionnaires already optimized for. Although currently serving a niche, innovations in electronic health records that incorporate PRO collection and other outcomes may eliminate the need for these collection platforms for the average clinician. Storing all of this data in a HIPAA compliant manner also presents a challenge. This is especially true for noncommercial systems which require professional set up and maintenance for a secure IT infrastructure. Besides that, encrypted external hard drives (e.g., IronKey™) and HIPAA-compliant cloud-based storage (e.g., Google Drive) can be considered other necessary equipment investments.

To facilitate high-quality data collection, consideration should also be given to hiring a full-time employee for day-to-day oversight. This can be in the form of research assistants, or medical assistants with minimal clinical duties, and is especially important for the academically geared practice where coordination may be a full-time endeavor. The outcomes assistant role is rooted in guiding patients through form completion and assuring patients get the proper questionnaires at certain timepoints. The assistant should also undertake the role of data input and organization, as well as basic analytics for comparison and preliminary statistics. Meanwhile, the physician needs to be the outcomes collection project champion. It is vital as the leader that the physician provides guidance for unordinary situations or outcomes, in addition to operational and financial oversight. Although largely "hands-off," this role requires availability for support.

Managing equipment and staff efficiently means developing an optimal routine with limited interruption of clinical care. Lessons learned from the FORCE-TJR, a joint replacement outcomes registry consisting of over 120 surgeons, indicate that patient PRO data should be available to the surgeon at the time of the patient encounter to provide the largest benefit to the care experience [42]. In this way, the surgeon can quantitatively assess physical function and pain while also saving time by only validating those results in the patient room rather than asking for an extensive history or update of the present illness. Remote data collection prior to the patient visit eliminates the burden of collecting outcomes in clinic and provides outcomes in advance of the patient encounter. Several outcome collection platforms and electronic health records have mechanisms to accomplish this, as discussed in the next section. Understandably, patients will not be 100% compliant with this and in-office systems need to be in place as a safety net. Harnessing the patients unused "waiting time" is key. To implement this successfully, we recommend a dedicated space to outcomes collection. It can be as simple as a private kiosk in the waiting area equipped with tablets, and the clerk/outcomes assistant there to facilitate the process. The patient can be instructed to do this at the registration desk just after registration. A general clinic flow diagram may help in the planning process for your practice (Fig. 9.2).

Collection Platforms

The recent emphasis on electronic collection in our modern healthcare system has spurred an increase in the number of available HIPAA-compliant electronic data capture systems. Currently, the most popular and commonly used electronic data collection systems in orthopedic surgery include OBERD, SOS, SOCRATES, and REDCap (Table 9.1).

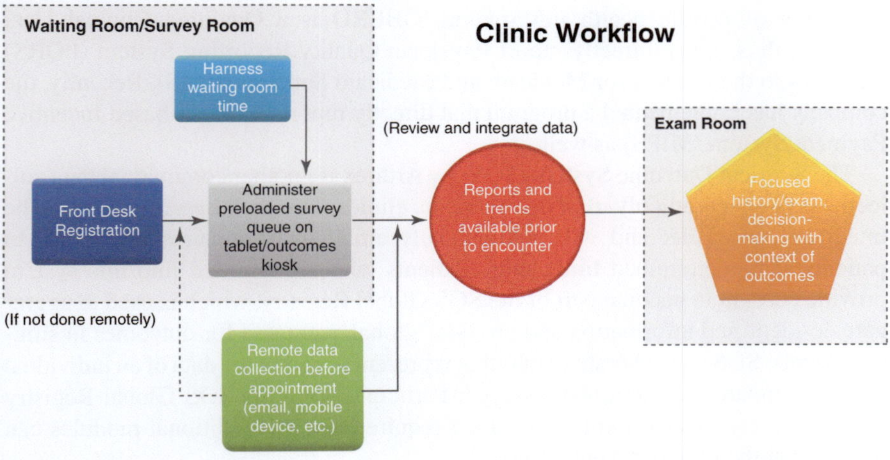

Fig. 9.2 An example of integrating outcomes collection into existing clinic workflow

Table 9.1 Electronic outcomes collection platforms

Electronic Data Capture System	OBERD	SOS	SOCRATES	REDCap
Vendor	Universal Research Solutions	Arthrex	Ortholink	Vanderbilt University
Commercial or Noncommercial	Commercial	Commercial	Commercial	Noncommercial
Security Measures	Centralized, encrypted storage	Centralized, encrypted storage	Dependent on local server	Dependent on local server
Integration with Electronic Health Records	Yes	Yes	No	No
Qualified Clinical Data Entry	Yes	No	No	No
Additional Features	Direct reporting of MIPS to CMS	Contribution to global registry, and comparison of individual patient scores to de-identified averages	Modules for anatomic-specific problems that can be further customized	Access to user-created, pre-built PROs in Consortium Library

The Outcomes-Based Electronic Research Database, otherwise known as OBERD, is an outcome data collection system developed and supported by Universal Research Solutions. Like all commercial products, OBERD requires a licensing agreement for use in clinic. OBERD can operate independent of electronic health record (EHR) systems, but is also capable of being integrated into them as well. Information received by OBERD is encrypted to ensure confidentiality and protection of private health information. OBERD is a Qualified Clinical Data Registry; thus, it can directly report Physician Quality Reporting System (PQRS) measures to the Centers for Medicare and Medicaid Services (CMS). Recently, the company has implemented a program that directly reports to Merit-based Incentive Payment System (MIPS) as well.

The Surgical Outcome System (SOS) by Arthrex is another commercial data collection system commonly used in orthopedic clinics. This web-based system can be integrated into EHR and will automatically email questionnaires and PROs to patients at predetermined timepoints. Patients who are enrolled into this system provide consent to become part of the SOS Global Registry, which is used to aggregate de-identified information and provide "global averages" for outcomes in similar patients. SOS can generate graphs that represent the outcome data of an individual patient compared to the global average. Participation in the SOS Global Registry requires an established minimum survey requirement, but additional modules can be added at the provider's preference.

SOCRATES (Standardised Orthopedic Clinical Research and Treatment Evaluation Software) is a commercial system by Ortholink Pty Ltd. Like the other commercial options, PROs can be collected within the clinic setting or remotely. These PROs come in preset modules that can be customized based on the provider's preference. Unlike OBERD and SOS, however, SOCRATES is established and operates within the local server of the clinical practice; that is, information collected from patients is stored locally and not by the commercial company. Thus, the security of private information relies on the protection offered by the local network. Currently, SOCRATES is not capable of integrating with clinical EHR.

The Research Electronic Data Capture, otherwise known as REDCap, is a secure, noncommercial, web-based application for building and managing surveys established by Vanderbilt University [43]. Although this data collection system is free for institutional partners, it requires contribution to the REDCap Consortium as well as significant local IT infrastructure and support. REDCap is protected and runs on the local server; however, it also communicates with Vanderbilt's server for specialized auto-scoring functionality. A unique feature of REDCap is the sharing of pre-built PROs and other forms within the Consortium Library. These PROs can be uploaded into projects for local use. Custom forms can also be built from scratch using various question types and instruments.

While we have highlighted these four electronic outcome collection systems, there are certainly many more commercial, noncommercial, and open source software available. Each of these platforms offers a variety of features, IT involvement, and costs. Thus, orthopedic providers should assess their own needs and choose the most appropriate platform for their own individual practice.

Final Considerations

There are a few "x-factors" worth mentioning that can be unaccounted for even in the most meticulously planned systems. Primarily, the patient represents the largest unpredictable factor, as they exert influence at every step of the data collection process. From their perspective, they receive a bombardment of forms to read, questions to answer, and signatures to give all while under duress from their issue that brings them to the office in the first place. Moreover, this process may be repeated at various other healthcare provider offices. Collectively, this defines the patient burden. Therefore, maintaining compliance is heavily reliant upon an upkeep of patient satisfaction. A balance exists between keeping question counts low while obtaining high quality, thorough data. Studies have shown that form length, number of words, and question counts all affect survey response rates [44–46]. Despite all of the research, an ideal threshold is hard to determine due to the heterogeneity of patient backgrounds, education, attentiveness that a provider is likely to come across. Computerized adaptive test forms can help lighten this burden, and keep outcomes collection short and focused.

The physician should also be invested in ensuring patient compliance. Oftentimes, the patient respects the doctor's opinion, and would be more amenable to completing forms if the surgeon personally assures the data's usefulness. One study has shown that patients are more than twice as likely to fill out health surveys if they know the organization/institution is conducting the study [47]. In a similar manner, knowing the physician is behind the reason for filling out questionnaires, rather than administrative initiatives, may give the patient a sense of importance behind recording their outcomes.

Registry Creation

To summarize, collecting clinical outcomes is becoming standard practice in medicine fueled by the transitions in medical policy and value-based reimbursements. Having a comprehensive approach will allow a surgical practice to create a patient registry rich with data concerning both objective and subjective outcomes. This information will prove useful for academic research, private practice overviews, and reimbursement leverage in contemporary payer schemes. Furthermore, the doctor–patient relationship will be enhanced as smooth outcomes collection can improve clinic efficiency, highlight the patient perspective, and trend clinical progress in real time for each office visit. Although a significant investment, thoughtful selection of outcomes, consideration of staff and equipment, and optimization of clinic flow for the typical patient will prove crucial for successful implementation.

References

1. Nwachukwu BU, Hamid KS, Bozic KJ. Measuring value in Orthopaedic surgery. JBJS Rev. 2013;1(1). p. ii.
2. Institute of Medicine (U.S.). Committee on Quality of Health Care in America. Crossing the quality chasm: a new health system for the 21st century. Washington D.C.: National Academy Press; 2001. xx. p. 337.
3. Kohn LT, Corrigan J, Donaldson MS. To err is human : building a safer health system. Washington DC: National Academy Press; 2000. xxi. p. 287.
4. Services CfMaM. Comprehensive Care for Joint Replacement Model Baltimore, MD2016 [updated December 21, 2016. Available from: https://innovation.cms.gov/initiatives/cjr.
5. Stark T, Walker B, Phillips JK, Fejer R, Beck R. Hand-held dynamometry correlation with the gold standard isokinetic dynamometry: a systematic review. PM R. 2011;3(5):472–9.
6. Hall JM, Azar FM, Miller RH, Smith R, Throckmorton TW. Accuracy and reliability testing of two methods to measure internal rotation of the glenohumeral joint. J Shoulder Elbow Surg. 2014;23(9):1296–300.
7. Dunn WR, Kuhn JE, Sanders R, An Q, Baumgarten KM, Bishop JY, et al. Symptoms of pain do not correlate with rotator cuff tear severity: a cross-sectional study of 393 patients with a symptomatic atraumatic full-thickness rotator cuff tear. J Bone Joint Surg Am. 2014;96(10):793–800.
8. Group MS, Unruh KP, Kuhn JE, Sanders R, An Q, Baumgarten KM, et al. The duration of symptoms does not correlate with rotator cuff tear severity or other patient-related features: a cross-sectional study of patients with atraumatic, full-thickness rotator cuff tears. J Shoulder Elbow Surg. 2014;23(7):1052–8.

9. Ryan M, Bisset L, Newsham-West R. Should we care about tendon structure? the disconnect between structure and symptoms in tendinopathy. J Orthop Sports Phys Ther. 2015;45(11):823–5.
10. Greenberg CC. Measuring outcomes in surgeryJohn L. Cameron AMC. Current surgical therapy. 11th ed: Elsevier Saunders; Philadelphia, PA 19103. 2014.
11. Deshpande PR, Rajan S, Sudeepthi BL, Abdul Nazir CP. Patient-reported outcomes: a new era in clinical research. Perspect Clin Res. 2011;2(4):137–44.
12. Hawkins RJ. Recommendations for evaluating and selecting appropriately valued outcome measures. Instr Course Lect. 2016;65:587–91.
13. AAOS. Information statement: principles of patient reported outcome measures (PROM) reporting: American Academy of Orthopaedic Surgeons; 2015 [Available from: http://www.aaos.org/uploadedFiles/PreProduction/About/Opinion_Statements/advistmt/1044%20Principles%20of%20Patient%20Reported%20Outcome%20Measures%20(PROMs)%20Reporting.pdf.
14. Mohtadi NG. Outcome measure development. Instr Course Lect. 2016;65:577–82.
15. Patel AA, Donegan D, Albert T. The 36-item short form. J Am Acad Orthop Surg. 2007;15(2):126–34.
16. Ware JE. User's manual for the SF-36v2 health survey. Quality Metric Inc.; Lincoln, RI 02865. 2nd ed; 2009. p. 309.
17. Webster KE, Feller JA. Use of the short form health surveys as an outcome measure for anterior cruciate ligament reconstruction. Knee Surg Sports Traumatol Arthrosc. 2014;22(5):1142–8.
18. Health R. KDQOL Frequently Asked Questions [What is the difference between the SF-36™ and the RAND-™?]. Available from: http://www.rand.org/health/surveys_tools/kdqol/faq.html.
19. Rabin R, de Charro F. EQ-5D: a measure of health status from the EuroQol Group. Ann Med. 2001;33(5):337–43.
20. Fryback DG, Dunham NC, Palta M, Hanmer J, Buechner J, Cherepanov D, et al. US norms for six generic health-related quality-of-life indexes from the National Health Measurement study. Med Care. 2007;45(12):1162–70.
21. University N. PROMIS: list of adult measures 2017 [Available from: http://www.healthmeasures.net/explore-measurement-systems/promis/intro-to-promis/list-of-adult-measures.
22. Witter JP. Introduction: PROMIS a first look across diseases. J Clin Epidemiol. 2016;73:87–8.
23. Wainer H, Dorans NJ, Flaugher R, Green BF, Mislevy RJ. Computerized adaptive testing: a primer: Routledge; New York, NY 10017. 2000.
24. Ardern CL, Osterberg A, Tagesson S, Gauffin H, Webster KE, Kvist J. The impact of psychological readiness to return to sport and recreational activities after anterior cruciate ligament reconstruction. Br J Sports Med. 2014;48(22):1613–9.
25. Ardern CL, Taylor NF, Feller JA, Whitehead TS, Webster KE. Psychological responses matter in returning to preinjury level of sport after anterior cruciate ligament reconstruction surgery. Am J Sports Med. 2013;41(7):1549–58.
26. Christino MA, Fleming BC, Machan JT, Shalvoy RM. Psychological factors associated with anterior cruciate ligament reconstruction recovery. Orthop J Sports Med. 2016;4(3):2325967116638341.
27. Brander V, Gondek S, Martin E, Stulberg SD. Pain and depression influence outcome 5 years after knee replacement surgery. Clin Orthop Relat Res. 2007;464:21–6.
28. Marks MR, Phillips D, Halsey DA, Wong A. Difficult conversations in Orthopaedics. Instr Course Lect. 2015;64:3–9.
29. Matava MJ, Howard DR, Polakof L, Brophy RH. Public perception regarding anterior cruciate ligament reconstruction. J Bone Joint Surg Am. 2014;96(10):e85.
30. Makhni EC, Padaki AS, Petridis PD, Steinhaus ME, Ahmad CS, Cole BJ, et al. High variability in outcome reporting patterns in high-impact ACL literature. J Bone Joint Surg Am. 2015;97(18):1529–42.
31. Marshall DA, Wasylak T, Khong H, Parker RD, Faris PD, Frank C. Measuring the value of total hip and knee arthroplasty: considering costs over the continuum of care. Clin Orthop Relat Res. 2012;470(4):1065–72.

32. Shirley ED, Sanders JO. Patient satisfaction: implications and predictors of success. J Bone Joint Surg Am. 2013;95(10):e69.
33. Graham B, Green A, James M, Katz J, Swiontkowski M. Measuring patient satisfaction in Orthopaedic surgery. J Bone Joint Surg Am. 2015;97(1):80–4.
34. Gill L, White L. A critical review of patient satisfaction. Leadersh Health Serv. 2009;22(1):8–19.
35. Baker PN, van der Meulen JH, Lewsey J, Gregg PJ, National Joint Registry for E, Wales. The role of pain and function in determining patient satisfaction after total knee replacement. Data from the National Joint Registry for England and Wales. J Bone Joint Surg Br. 2007;89(7):893–900.
36. Kwon SK, Kang YG, Kim SJ, Chang CB, Seong SC, Kim TK. Correlations between commonly used clinical outcome scales and patient satisfaction after total knee arthroplasty. J Arthroplasty. 2010;25(7):1125–30.
37. Lim JB, Chou AC, Yeo W, Lo NN, Chia SL, Chin PL, et al. Comparison of patient quality of life scores and satisfaction after common Orthopaedic surgical interventions. Eur J Orthop Surg Traumatol. 2015;25(6):1007–12.
38. Henn RF, Ghomrawi H, Rutledge JR, Mazumdar M, Mancuso CA, Marx RG. Preoperative patient expectations of total shoulder arthroplasty. J Bone Joint Surg Am. 2011;93(22):2110–5.
39. Mancuso CA, Jout J, Salvati EA, Sculco TP. Fulfillment of patients' expectations for total hip arthroplasty. J Bone Joint Surg Am. 2009;91(9):2073–8.
40. Jackson JL, Chamberlin J, Kroenke K. Predictors of patient satisfaction. Soc Sci Med. 2001;52(4):609–20.
41. Roberts N, Bradley B, Williams D. Use of SMS and tablet computer improves the electronic collection of elective Orthopaedic patient reported outcome measures. Ann R Coll Surg Engl. 2014;96(5):348–51.
42. Ayers DC, Zheng H, Franklin PD. Integrating patient-reported outcomes into Orthopaedic clinical practice: proof of concept from FORCE-TJR. Clin Orthop Relat Res. 2013;471(11):3419–25.
43. Harris PA, Taylor R, Thielke R, Payne J, Gonzalez N, Conde JG. Research electronic data capture (REDCap)--a metadata-driven methodology and workflow process for providing translational research informatics support. J Biomed Inform. 2009;42(2):377–81.
44. Edwards P, Roberts I, Clarke M, DiGuiseppi C, Pratap S, Wentz R, et al. Increasing response rates to postal questionnaires: systematic review. BMJ. 2002;324(7347):1183.
45. Jepson C, Asch DA, Hershey JC, Ubel PA. In a mailed physician survey, questionnaire length had a threshold effect on response rate. J Clin Epidemiol. 2005;58(1):103–5.
46. McFarlane E, Olmsted MG, Murphy J, Hill CA. Nonresponse bias in a mail survey of physicians. Eval Health Prof. 2007;30(2):170–85.
47. Beebe TJ, Jenkins SM, Anderson KJ, Davern ME. Survey-related experiential and attitudinal correlates of future health survey participation: results of a statewide survey. Mayo Clin Proc. 2008;83(12):1358–63.

Chapter 10
Pursuing a Dual Degree

Eric C. Makhni

On Pursuing an MBA (Or Any Other Secondary Professional Degree)

The goal of this book is to introduce you to some of the fundamental concepts of practice management *without* the need to go out and get an MBA. That being said, dual degrees are still quite powerful, especially if they are obtained with a specific purpose in mind. With the popularity of advanced, non-clinical degrees for healthcare professionals, there has been a number of different types of secondary degrees available. The question then becomes, "*Should I get a second degree?*" This chapter will summarize the utility of a second degree for physicians. While most attention will be paid to the MBA (as it is the most commonly sought second degree), there are numerous other dual-degree options that will be introduced.

As a medical student, I was fortunate to be at the right place and the right time, when the dual MD-MBA degree program was just beginning. Traditionally, a full-time MBA consists of two academic years of coursework, allowing a summer in between for internships. At the time (and it is not much different even today), students in the MD-MBA track spent their first 3 years in medical school, their fourth year in a dedicated MBA curriculum, and their fifth year in a combination of both the MD program and the MBA program. In order to make up that half-year of coursework we missed from the business school, we performed various courses in the first 2 years of medical school along with a number of different scholarly projects through the 5 years. The program has become so popular in the ensuing years that the number of applications into the program greatly outnumbered the available spots, making it increasingly challenging to matriculate in.

E. C. Makhni
Division of Sports Medicine, Department of Orthopedic Surgery, Henry Ford Health System, West Bloomfield, MI, USA

E. C. Makhni et al. (eds.), *Orthopedic Practice Management*,
https://doi.org/10.1007/978-3-319-96938-1_10

Why a Dual Degree?

As you will see throughout this book, a successful career in modern medicine is only partly due to your actual clinical or surgical skills. Most of your success in building a practice, being a successful leader, or being an effective administrator is based upon a skillset that – amazingly – is ignored throughout coursework in medical school and residency training. And so, your option is to either (a) learn it on your own, (b) learn it through trial and error, or (c) obtain a secondary degree that will teach you some of these principles (you will still have to do plenty of (a) and (b), however!).

The idea that physicians must be trained in business matters is not new. In fact, in 1987, Dr. John Bernard Henry published a letter to the editor in JAMA calling for dual MD-MBA training for aspiring physician-leaders [1]. In a recent study by professors from my MD-MBA program [2], study authors found that students in the dual MD-MBA degree, compared to peers in the traditional medical school program, were relatively similar with regards to medical school performance and pre-medical school testing metrics. Those who pursued the dual degree reported a desire to either further personal professional interests or make an impact on healthcare delivery and/or administration. Most interestingly, however, was the fact that all students in the program reported a commitment to beginning and completing a clinical residency. Therefore, most students pursuing a dual degree actually do want to become physician-leaders, as opposed to those business leaders with medical backgrounds.

Getting a second degree while already completing the MD is a very convenient option. For one, you are already in school, and therefore there is no need to interrupt clinical residency or practice. You are also already in “student mode” and have no problem continuing with more required reading, homework, and tests. For most of our readers, however, you may already be in practice, with clinical and personal responsibilities that will most definitely preclude you from embarking on a 2-year academic adventure. The opportunity cost would simply be too high. Or, also equally likely, your medical school did not have a joint degree. Additionally, you may have only realized just recently that a second degree would be pretty helpful, as you discover the hurdles you deal with on a daily basis have little, if any, to do with actual clinical medicine.

The question then becomes – is it too late to get a second degree? If not, what degree, and what program, is reasonable to pursue while not abandoning your clinical practice (and family!)?

Types of Second Degrees: Options Abound

Before even contemplating pursuit of a second degree – whether still in medical school or a seasoned practitioner – you must first ask yourself “*Why?*”. *Why* do you need that second degree? What skill are you hoping to develop? What challenge are you looking to overcome? What are your ultimate career goals? The answer to these questions will guide you as to whether or not a second degree is for you, and if so, which degree to pursue.

As I mentioned earlier, it may be extremely challenging to leave your current situation and pursue a full-time dual degree, especially one that requires more than 1 year of full-time coursework. This may be possible to do if you are still a resident, and I have many colleagues that have gone down this route in the middle of residency or just prior to fellowship. Fortunately, there are a number of different options for second degrees that are more flexible in structure, allowing you to continue with your practice while completing requisite coursework.

Common Degree Types

MBA

The MBA – or Master of Business Administration – is by far the most common and well-known dual-degree option for aspiring physician-leaders. A traditional degree is 2 years long; however, numerous variations exist. In a typical MBA, the curriculum consists of a core set of coursework along with elective courses that tailor to the student's individual career or personal interests. Examples of basic coursework include principles of finance, accounting, economics, organizational behavior, leadership, negotiations, and ethics. Each school has a different take on how to organize this required core set of courses, and not all schools require students take a core curriculum. But, for aspiring physician-leaders, these common disciplines should be covered in the least.

The advantage of most MBA programs is that they allow the students to spend at least some part of their coursework in classes that are tailored to the career goals of the student. One must remember that a vast majority of traditional MBA students have taken some time off between completing college and starting an MBA program. Therefore, students already have developed some "real-world" skills and furthermore have an idea of their specific career aspirations. This allows them to tailor their course curriculum, internships, and scholastic activities in business school toward their ultimate career goals. For instance, if a student comes from an investment banking background and wants to further his/her career in finance, they will likely focus on advanced coursework in finance theory, investments, venture capital, private equity, and so forth. Similarly, those looking to pursue a career in marketing will ignore those courses and pursue coursework in marketing, consumer goods, etc.

The MBA is very practical for physicians because it provides not only the fundamental coursework but also multiple options for courses and activities that are directly relevant to pursuing a career in healthcare administration or leadership. The core curriculum will equip the physician-student with the fundamental concepts and language needed to participate in business matters in the healthcare setting.

It is very difficult to lead a large multi-specialty practice or department if you do not comprehend the most basic tenets of marketing, supply chain management, leadership, and organizational behavior. Moreover, the MBA allows the physician-student to pursue focused coursework specialized to healthcare. This may entail healthcare administration, healthcare innovation, advanced topics in leadership and management, and the like. *This is precisely why it is so important to understand your career goals before starting your advanced degree. If you aspire to spend your career in device innovation and entrepreneurship, it would be a colossal waste if you leave business school without taking coursework in innovation, patents, venture capital, private equity,* etc. *Similarly, if you want to be a hospital administrator, these same courses may be useless to you. Alternatively, if you don't think about your career goals, you will graduate taking a random smattering of classes that may or may not have any impact on your future work.*

One of the main advantages of the MBA, in my humble opinion, is the opportunity to think of the world around you in a *macroscopic* perspective. Throughout undergraduate and medical school, along with residency and fellowship, physicians spend most of our time considering *microscopic* issues. What medication best treats condition X? Where should I put my graft for the perfect ACL? How many screws does this fracture need for a stable repair construct? All of these issues are largely very small in scope, affecting one part of one organ system for one patient. Let us think about the alternative.

In business school (or any similar post-graduate discipline), attention is largely placed on macroscopic issues. How does a supply chain error in inventory cause a downstream effect on operating room productivity? How does a delay of 2 weeks construction on a new project cause millions of dollars in lost revenue? How does ineffective communication and suboptimal office environment create a department-wide culture of mediocrity and poor results?

In addition to being forced to think of the world, and healthcare in particular, on a large scale, the MBA truly helps physicians consider multiple stakeholders in future business decisions. Rarely does one action have *no* impact on something else. Giving one more day of operating room block time to Dr. X means that Dr. Y gets 1 day less, and so on and so on. Such teaching also helps the physician understand that climbing the professional ladder has so *little* to do with his/her skills in the clinic or operating room and so *much* to do with his/her skills in the boardroom. If you fight with everyone to get your way in the short term, you will likely hinder most of your long-term aspirations. While these examples may seem common sense, we have all seen peers and superiors blindly abandon these basic tenets of business success and then act surprised when their careers fail to progress as they like.

MPH

The MPH – or Master of Public Health – is another degree that is very commonly pursued by healthcare professionals. It is also a very common degree that is obtained during medical school. At its core, the MPH focuses on public health, focusing on delivery of care both from a domestic and international perspective. Within the confines of population-based healthcare also lies coursework in statistics and epidemiology. These courses can be invaluable to those focusing on a career in clinical research. However, for most researchers, collaboration with those skilled in biostatistics is usually sufficient enough. Additional coursework is dedicated to healthcare administration, occupational medicine, and other social aspects related to healthcare delivery. When combined with a medical degree, joint MD-MPH programs can be completed within the 4 years required for the MD (such as through summer curricula) or with the addition of one extra year.

MHSA

The MHSA – Master of Health Services Administration – is a relatively new degree program with obvious applications to healthcare professionals. This program is not just for physicians, but is also relevant for all professionals working in the healthcare industry. Unlike the MPH, most MHSA programs are focused on healthcare delivery in the United States. Like the MBA, the MHSA can be completed in a traditional 2-year format, but alternative formats (more on this below) also exist.

The best way to understand the goal of a particular MHSA program is to study its curriculum. For example, the sample curriculum from the University of Michigan MHSA program (https://sph.umich.edu/hmp/programs/mhsa.html) [3] includes coursework that can be found in most MBA programs (organizational theory, professional development), along with those tailored to healthcare delivery (health services, healthcare accounting, healthcare policy), and even some coursework from an MPH program (statistics and epidemiology, environmental health sciences). Therefore, the MHSA may present a unique opportunity to pursue a very healthcare-focused curriculum in preparation for a successful career in healthcare administration and leadership.

Executive Education Programs

Another attractive option for obtaining a second degree is through executive education. The difference with many "Exec Ed" programs and traditional degree programs is that students in Exec Ed are typically already executives. Many are leaders of their companies, firms, divisions, or departments who are looking to get training in a very specific skillset in business education. For example, Harvard Business School offers several different types of exec ed. programs, and their selection can be seen at https://www.exed.hbs.edu/programs/Pages/default.aspx [4].

Unlike traditional degree programs, these immersions can vary in length and timing. Typically, they are shorter in length (spanning 2–3 weeks) and more intensive, thus acting as a true immersion. Physicians who are mid-career or are already in a leadership track may benefit tremendously from these programs.

Do I Need to Have 2 Years to Do One of These Degrees?

The answer to the above question is yes…and no. Traditional programs at many academic institutions will treat these degrees like degrees from other departments, in that they require students to be full-time students on a traditional full-time academic calendar. However, there are many opportunities for clinicians to complete this coursework in flexible ways.

Flexibility comes with respect to both coursework dissemination and scheduling. With the popularity of online education, many schools (and even top academic institutions) offer programs in an online format. These include full degrees for the MBA, MHSA, and MPH, as well as other types of healthcare degrees. Such a program is ideal for the physician who has little flexibility in traveling to a campus for their degree, be it for personal or professional reasons.

As the online format allows for increased flexibility, programs are also offering unique structures to in-classroom learning. Multiple programs offer weekend-only courses, or scheduled courses interspersed throughout the year. These options are especially attractive if the campus is close to your practice, such that you would not have to travel a significant distance to attend your courses.

Thanks to the popularity of many of these programs, you will surely be able to find a program that fits your interests and logistical freedom (or constraints). From a financial perspective, these programs can be quite expensive. It is important to explore creative ways to finance the education. If the hospital or department is encouraging you to attend these courses, and certainly if they are hoping to benefit from your newfound skillset, they may be willing to support the cost of tuition as well as the time for lost clinical productivity. If you are in a practice in which there is no such infrastructure to fund your tuition, then a simple cost-benefit analysis will help guide you which degree is most suitable.

References

1. Henry JB. MD-MBA: a dual degree whose time has come. JAMA. 1987;257(13):1727–8.
2. Krupat E, Dienstag JL, Kester WC, Finkelstein SN. Medical students who pursue a joint MD/MBA degree: who are they and where are they heading? Eval Health Prof. 2016 pii: 0163278715620831. [Epub ahead of print].
3. University of Michigan MHSA curriculum program. Available at: https://sph.umich.edu/hmp/programs/mhsa.html.
4. Harvard Business School Executive Education programs. Available at: https://www.exed.hbs.edu/programs/Pages/default.aspx.

Chapter 11
Healthcare Policy

Ramin M. Lalezari and Christopher J. Dy

Introduction

The design and implementation of health policies drive the manner in which we deliver healthcare. Although these policies strive to balance quality and expense, in 2000, the World Health Organization ranked the United States healthcare system 31st for quality and 1st for expenditure [1]. The discrepancy between spending and quality of care in the United States is a persistent subject of political debate, leading to a number of reforms and reform proposals. Before discussing the current state of health policy in this country, however, it is important to understand the context and the history from which it has evolved.

A History of Healthcare in the United States

Prior to 1929, medical care in the United States was financed entirely out-of-pocket, save for injuries suffered on the job. In the early twentieth century, healthcare costs began to increase beyond what an individual could afford. This, combined with the unpredictability of the need for future care, was an impetus to design a system in which Americans could insure their medical costs. Health insurance was first offered

R. M. Lalezari
Washington University School of Medicine, Department of Orthopedic Surgery, St. Louis, MO, USA
e-mail: rlalezari@wustl.edu

C. J. Dy (✉)
Washington University School of Medicine, Department of Orthopedic Surgery, Division of Hand and Upper Extremity Surgery, Department of Surgery, Division of Public Health Sciences, St. Louis, MO, USA
e-mail: dyc@wudosis.wustl.edu

E. C. Makhni et al. (eds.), *Orthopedic Practice Management*,
https://doi.org/10.1007/978-3-319-96938-1_11

in the United States in 1929, with the conception of Blue Cross by Justin F. Kimball to insure teachers against hospital care costs at Baylor University Hospital [2]. Soon, the plans spread to other single-hospital systems, and then expanded to cover multiple hospitals. Eventually, Blue Shield was developed by the California Medical Association to begin covering physician fees as well.

During the Second World War, wage freezes left employers struggling to find ways to attract employees outside of salary increases. Around that same time, the Internal Revenue Code was amended to allow deduction of employer-paid health insurance, creating a tax incentive to implement such programs. As a result, employer-issued health insurance became an increasingly large portion of coverage by the end of the war. Over the next two decades, the US government became concerned with the large numbers of both the poor and the elderly who lacked health insurance coverage. By 1965, President Lyndon Johnson implemented the Medicare program to cover health expenditures for citizens older than the age of 65, as well as the Medicaid program to do the same for those below certain income thresholds. While Medicare became financed and implemented on a federal level, the operation of Medicaid was left to the states.

After the enactment of those programs, healthcare expenditures ballooned. In the 5 years between 1966 and 1971, national health expenditures climbed to nearly triple the rate of the consumer price index (a common measure of inflation) [3]. In response, Congress passed the Health Maintenance Organizations Act of 1973, centering US health policy on the managed care model. The act greatly expanded the number of Health Maintenance Organizations (HMOs), which gained popularity for the way they shifted physician reimbursements away from the fee-for-service model. The implications of this shift in principles were far-reaching and will be explored later in this chapter.

Financing Healthcare in the United States

Why Health Insurance?

Why is it that to pay for healthcare, consumers demand insurance? Insurance allows individuals to forego income today in order to shield themselves from expenditures at a later date. It is the uncertainty about the future that creates a desire for that protection. Thus, individuals pool money together by paying insurance premiums such that one entity (i.e., the insurance company) is able to bear the brunt of the cost when an unexpected medical expense occurs for a beneficiary.

To fully appreciate the complexities of the US healthcare system, it is important to understand the economics of health insurance. If we think like economists for a moment and assume that people act rationally, there is no incentive for an individual to invest more money (via insurance premiums) into their health insurance than his or her average annual expenditure. Although it is difficult for an individual to predict his or her average annual expenditure, insurance actuaries are able to predict these expenditures for an entire beneficiary pool. Economic principles predict that the market would bid premiums down to equal the aggregate average annual expenditure for the entire beneficiary pool. If this occurred, the insurance company's profits would be zero. Given the profits generated by insurance companies, these economic principles are not born out, largely due to individual attitudes toward risk. In general, the magnitude of "happiness" gained from receiving a dollar of income is smaller than the magnitude of "unhappiness" lost from losing a dollar of income. This concept is referred to as "risk aversion." As an example, imagine a coin flip game in which the outcome of "heads" wins $100, whereas the outcome of "tails" loses $100. The average, or expected, outcome of this game is walking away with nothing, yet due to risk aversion, the average person would pay to avoid playing this game. In the context of insurance, beneficiaries are effectively paying a surcharge to the insurance company to avoid the bad outcome of losing money to a large medical expenditure; this imbalance generates profit for the insurance company. Furthermore, insurance plans enable individuals to pool their own individual risk for medical expenditure, reducing the effect of outlier events among all beneficiaries.

Ultimately, this fear of uncertainty and aversion to risk drives the existence of a market for insuring health. In the United States, this market is comprised of these main categories: Medicare, Medicaid, employer-provided private insurance, consumer-purchased private insurance, and other public programs (State Children's Health Insurance Program, Veteran's Health Administration, Indian Health Service, etc.) (Fig. 11.1). Beyond this, there are 29 million Americans who are uninsured [4] and have been the target of recent reform efforts.

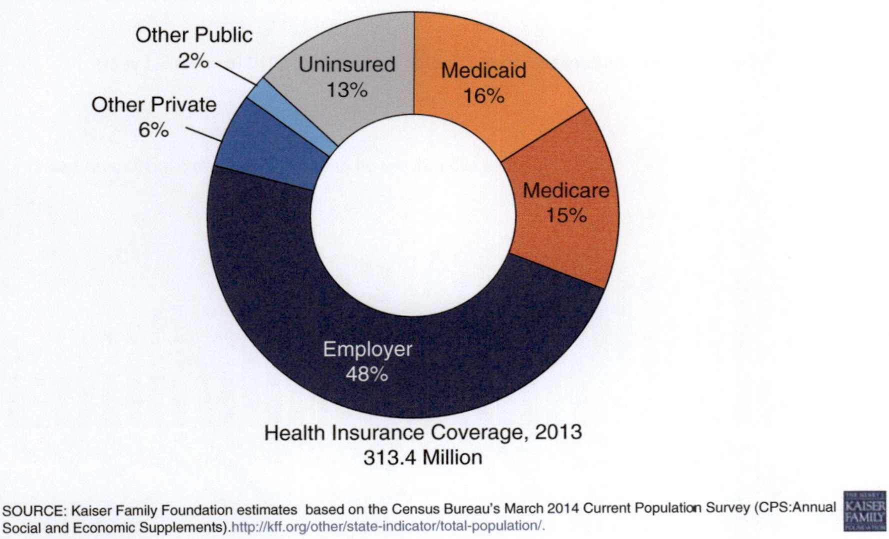

Fig. 11.1 Types of insurance coverage in the United States [5]. Breakdown, by percentage of Americans covered, of the different types of health insurance coverage in the United States. "Other Public" refers to governmental insurance programs other than Medicare and Medicaid, such as the State Children's Health Insurance Program (CHIP) or the Indian Health Service. "Other Private" refers to any insurance purchased by the beneficiary, rather than his/her employer, from private companies. (Reprinted from Ref. [5])

Healthcare Reform

Impetus for Healthcare Reform

In 2010, the United States spent 18% of its Gross Domestic Product (GDP) on healthcare. That translates to a per capita spend of $8233, the highest among countries within the Organization for Economic Co-operation and Development (OECD) (Fig. 11.2). This increased expenditure is not necessarily associated with higher quality of care: In fact, a 2006 study found a negative correlation between increased Medicare spending and 1-year survival after myocardial infarction [6]. The World Health Organization ranks the United States 31st in life expectancy, 44th in infant mortality, and 44th in mortality rates for noncommunicable diseases, despite the high national health expenditure [7]. In addition, one out of every six nonelderly Americans remained uninsured in 2010 [8]. These statistics provide the context for healthcare reform during Barack Obama's first term.

The Overhaul

When Obama took office in 2008, he made clear that health reform would be a major focus of his administration. Taking lessons from a failed healthcare reform effort during the administration of Bill Clinton, he enlisted White House Chief of

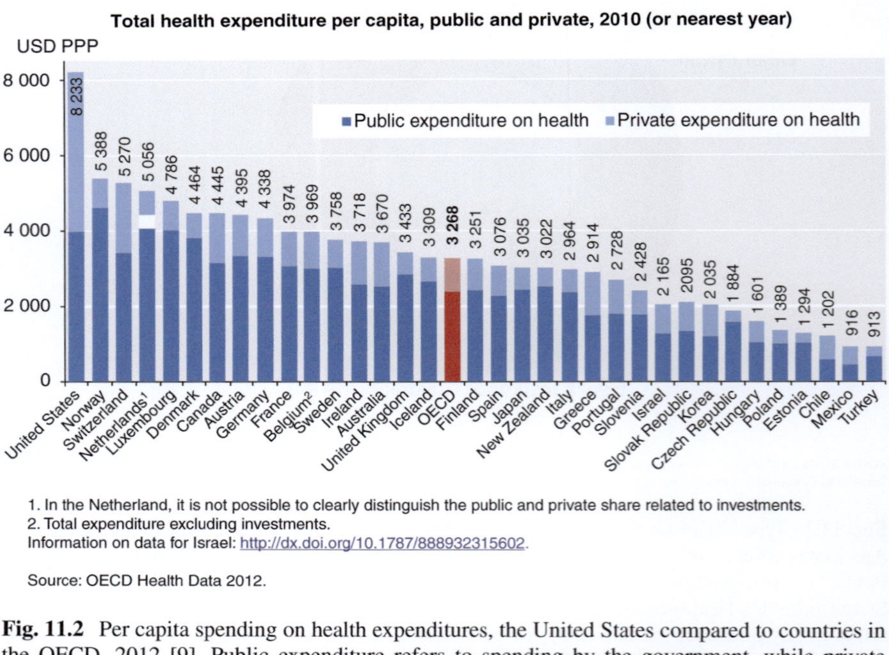

Fig. 11.2 Per capita spending on health expenditures, the United States compared to countries in the OECD, 2012 [9]. Public expenditure refers to spending by the government, while private expenditure refers to spending by citizens. The United States has a similar per capita public expenditure, while its private expenditure is significantly higher. (Reprinted from Kane [9])

Staff Rahm Emanuel to unify the houses of Congress behind a comprehensive healthcare reform bill. Jonathan Gruber, a health economist from MIT who designed Massachusetts' health reform legislation under then-governor Mitt Romney 2 years prior, was a key advisor to Obama's reform effort, and included many of the provisions that had been successful in Massachusetts. Interest groups, too, were brought into the discussions this time, leading to support of health reform from Pharmaceutical Research and Manufacturers of America (PhRMA), the American Medical Association (AMA), and the American Hospital Association (AHA). After a number of contentious committee battles, the Affordable Care Act (ACA) passed the House of Representatives 220–207 and the Senate 56–43, and was signed into law by President Obama on March 30, 2010.

Key Provisions

The Exchanges

The ACA introduced government-run health insurance exchange markets over the Internet in all 50 states. States are allowed to manage their own exchanges, but if they decline, the federal government will operate it. These exchanges were designed to be competitive marketplaces for insurance plans to be bought and sold. The government's rationale for such a marketplace is that a competitive marketplace would create pressure for premiums to be bid downward. The online interface has the additional advantage of displaying pricing and plan benefits in a format that is easy for the user to understand and compare.

Coverage

After passage of the ACA, there were new coverage requirements for all health insurance plans offered. There are currently 12 categories of required services and benefits (Table 11.1). Of these, the category of "preventative and wellness services" is to be

Table 11.1 Required coverage of services and benefits by insurance plans post-ACA

Ambulatory patient services
Emergency services
Hospitalization
Pregnancy, maternity, and newborn care
Mental health and substance use disorder services
Prescription drugs
Rehabilitative and habilitative services and devices
Laboratory services
Preventative and wellness services and chronic disease management
Pediatric services, including oral and vision care
Birth control coverage
Breastfeeding coverage

provided with no cost-sharing mechanisms on the side of the consumer. This was implemented to incentivize beneficiaries to engage in preventative care without the concern for financial barriers, in order to attempt to control long-term healthcare costs.

Another significant coverage change was that insurers can no longer deny coverage to an individual with a preexisting condition, nor can they raise premiums or cancel coverage because of claims made. The only health status question that can affect the rates charged is smoking status. In addition, the law implemented a medical loss provision dictating that insurance plans had to keep their "medical loss ratios" above 80%. The medical loss ratio is the percentage of premiums collected that are actually paid toward claims. In 2011, insurers paid over a billion dollars in rebates to beneficiaries in order to comply with this provision [10].

These provisions sparked a number of controversies in the years following passage of the ACA. Most of them centered on the coverage requirements. In 2011, the US Preventative Service Task Force (USPSTF) announced what preventative services were to be included in the "preventative and wellness services" category. Religious groups opposed the inclusion of contraceptive coverage in those benefit requirements. This led to an exemption for religious organizations providing coverage for their employees, through which they could opt out of providing contraceptive benefits.

There has also been debate around the requirement for minimum benefits across all beneficiaries. For example, males and postmenopausal women are still covered for "Pregnancy, maternity, and newborn care." Opponents argue that individuals should be able to select the benefits that they desire in their plans to reduce their individual premiums. Proponents of the current setup maintain that women of reproductive age should not be penalized in their premiums, the same way that those with preexisting conditions are not penalized.

Insuring the 17%

One of the key goals of the healthcare reform effort was to insure the 17% of Americans that remained uninsured in 2010 [8]. Not only were reformers attempting to increase access to healthcare for all Americans, but it was also noted that of those 50 million uninsured, there was a disproportionate number of young adults aged 18–34. Forty percent of the uninsured represented this age demographic, despite them making up 25% of the population (Fig. 11.3). Now, one might argue that these individuals, being healthier and therefore less likely to utilize their health insurance, do not always need to carry coverage. However, this instigates a commonly understood economic problem in the insurance market known as *adverse selection*.

If we take a step back to a more fundamental understanding of how insurance works, we can see how this problem arises. To simplify, suppose that the only cost to a beneficiary to purchase insurance is the premium. Insurance actuaries model and predict the average healthcare expenditure for an individual, build in a markup for risk aversion, and charge that amount as a premium. Suppose that amount is $1000; for this example, we will ignore the markup for risk aversion. This should

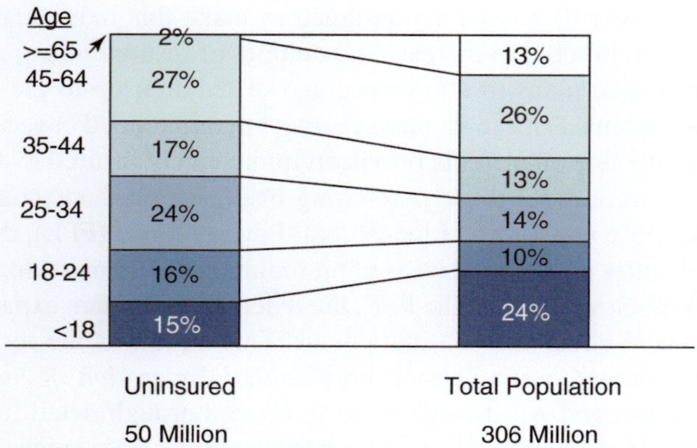

Note: Totals may not sum to 100% due to rounding.
Source: U.S. Census Bureau, *Income Poverty and Health Insurance Coverage in the United States: 2010, 2011.*

Fig. 11.3 Profile of the uninsured vs. total population by age, 2010 [11]. (Reprinted from [11])

result in a break-even for insurance companies, regardless of the number of individuals that enroll in the plan. An issue arises, though, from the fact that there is an asymmetry of information between the insurance company and the beneficiary. The beneficiaries know more about their own health status, and their own propensity to incur medical expenses, than the insurance company does. Thus, only those individuals who expect to incur more annual expenditure than the premium – more than $1000 – would enroll, which means that to cover these expenditures, the insurance company would need to raise the premium above the average individual expenditure for the entire population, say to $1500. But this would cause the individuals who expect to incur between $1000 and $1500 to decline purchasing the plan, and the insurance company is left with only a pool of individuals expecting to incur at least $1500. As this continues, premiums rise, while the insurance pool narrows to only the costliest of beneficiaries. This is the problem of adverse selection.

Together, adverse selection and the desire to increase access to healthcare prompted the ACA's individual mandate. Under this provision, individuals would be required to carry health insurance or pay a tax penalty. Once fully phased in, this penalty will equal the greater of $695 or 2.5% of taxable income. Such a requirement was included in the failed reform efforts by President Clinton, and was also a big feature of the Romneycare plan in Massachusetts. The individual mandate became a focal point of debate around the ACA when 25 states, along with the National Federation of Independent Businesses, filed a lawsuit against the Department of Health and Human Services in 2011. The suit argued that under the Commerce Clause of the US Constitution, individuals could not be made to purchase a good or service by the federal government. *National Federation of Independent Businesses v. Sebelius* rose to the US Supreme Court, who in a 5–4 landmark decision, ruled that the penalties implemented by the individual mandate were a valid exercise of Congress' taxing power.

There were a number of provisions designed to make this individual mandate more attainable. First, in a bid to increase the number of insured young adults, the ACA required insurance plans to allow coverage of children up to the age of 26 under their parents' plans. Prior to its passage, most plans stopped covering dependent children after the age of 21. This provision immediately insured over 700,000 young adults [12]. Second, for those purchasing insurance on the exchanges with incomes between 133% and 400% of the Federal Poverty Level (FPL), the government provided subsidies to offset the costs of premiums on a sliding scale. Third, for those with incomes below 133% of the FPL, the federal government expanded state Medicaid programs to cover all such individuals. This topic was the second piece debated in the Supreme Court's hearing on *National Federation of Independent Businesses v. Sebelius*, and will be discussed in more thorough detail later in this chapter. Lastly, the ACA expanded employer-based insurance coverage through an employer mandate.

The ACA enacted a requirement for businesses with 50 or more full-time employees to offer health insurance as an employment benefit or face a penalty. These plans must cover a minimum of 60% of the cost of services, and be available for less than 9.5% of the employee's annual income. The law defines full-time employees as those working for at least 120 days/year and at least 30 hours/week. For small businesses with less than 50 employees, the government offers tax credits to subsidize the cost of insuring their employees, along with a separate health insurance exchange program for them to pool their employees together and negotiate better rates. Opponents of these employer provisions argue that for small businesses, premiums can become expensive because the pool of employees is smaller. A smaller pool means less sharing of risk, and thus a riskier and more expensive package of employees to cover. Others argued that the full-time employee definition would lead to manipulation by employers to fall beneath those thresholds by involuntarily changing full-time employees to part-time. Whether or not labor practices have changed as a result of the ACA has remained questionable [13].

The Future of the ACA and Healthcare Reform

Almost immediately after its signing, the ACA received strong backlash from Republican lawmakers calling for its repeal and filing bills to do so as soon as the very next day. Opposition to the ACA led to at least 60 more votes to repeal, a number of drawn-out legal battles, and a governmental shutdown in 2013. Never has the prospect of repeal been more real than after the election of Donald Trump. His campaign vowed to repeal the reform bill within the first 100 days of taking office. As of this writing, the administration's intention remains unclear on whether that will occur. But along with Republican lawmakers controlling both houses of Congress and a Supreme Court soon to sway the same way, changes are imminent. Rather than attempt to summarize the many proposed alternatives to the ACA, the remainder of this section will attempt to address a number of provisions that characterize the Republican alternatives to the ACA. All proposed alternatives would repeal at least part of the ACA, with near consensus on repeal of the individual mandate. In the following sections, we discuss provisions that are often included in Republican-sponsored health reform bills.

Tax Credits for Insurance Premiums

Republican lawmakers agree that financial assistance from the government is required to make health insurance affordable. Where the ACA provides individuals with subsidies to fund health insurance premiums, Republican plans incorporate tax credits. The main difference is that the ACA subsidies are tied to an individual's income, such that the financial benefits decrease as income rises. This gives relatively more support to lower income individuals to purchase insurance. The tax credits included in Republican plans would provide flat tax benefits regardless of income level. These are controversial due to the higher dollar amount of the benefit given to those in higher tax brackets, along with the fact that those who do not have an income would receive no assistance at all. It is estimated that such tax credits would lead to an increase in the number of the uninsured by 15.6 million, despite decreases in the uninsured rate for high-income individuals [14].

Health Savings Accounts

A Health Savings Account (HSA) is an account in which individuals can deposit funds to be used for medical expenses. These accounts are offered alongside "high-deductible health plans" (HDHPs). HDHPs offer lower premiums to beneficiaries in exchange for higher *deductibles* – the amount of total healthcare expenditures that the beneficiary must pay before any insurance payments kick in. HSAs are not subject to tax liabilities, and neither are the payments made from them. They are designed to encourage individuals to save a portion of their income for their own medical expenses, similar to the intended function of insurance premiums. The funds distributed into an HSA roll over from year-to-year, unlike related Flexible Savings Accounts (FSAs). A number of Republican healthcare plans advocate expansion of HSAs by allowing larger contributions and extending what types of payments can be covered through an HSA. They contend that HSAs allow individuals more freedom in determining how much they pay for their care. In addition, having the beneficiary bear more of the cost of care might reduce the incentive to overutilize care. Opponents argue that HSAs disproportionately benefit the young and healthy, shifting the burden of cost on the rest of the population. Furthermore, there is concern that while HSAs may prevent overutilization of services, they may go too far by leading individuals to delay necessary care. While some individuals might reduce their spending by switching from brand name drugs to generics, others might instead avoid critical care [15].

Medicaid Block Grants

Some health reform proposals promote the use of block grants as an alternative to the current Medicaid structure. Rather than a joint financial effort by state and federal governments to support Medicaid, block grants would distribute the federal funds directly to states for them to run their Medicaid programs as they see fit. Medicaid remains a state-operated program, and states have already begun to experiment with a variety of implementations. A large portion of this experimentation has been with the managed care model of healthcare delivery, described in detail later in this chapter. States have been contracting with private managed care organizations, which employ a variety of cost-cutting strategies, to operate their Medicaid programs. Medicaid managed care has become quite popular – since the turn of the millennium, the percentage of Medicaid enrollees covered by a managed care plan increased from 56% to 74% [16]. Replacement of expanded Medicaid programs with block grants would likely further popularize the use of the managed care model to operate Medicaid among the states. Supporters believe that these changes would significantly reduce overall Medicaid costs and allow states more freedom to conduct their programs. However, this would likely lead to cuts in eligibility and levels of care for the Medicaid population.

High-Risk Pooling

Prior to the ACA, individuals with preexisting conditions were often turned away from traditional health insurance plans. To combat this, 35 states had implemented *high-risk pools* to fill the gap. These states' governments would finance policies for these individuals who were deemed "high-risk," and thus expensive to cover. Passage of the ACA made these pools obsolete by preventing insurance companies from denying coverage due to preexisting conditions. A repeal of the ACA, though, would reintroduce that gap in care. While some alternative plans do maintain the provision that those with preexisting conditions not be turned away, they are less feasible without an individual mandate to balance adverse selection with healthy individuals.

Thus, many proposed alternative plans advocate reintroduction of high-risk pooling. Such pooling would reduce premium amounts for those outside of the pools, since healthy individuals' premiums would no longer be used to subsidize those with preexisting conditions. However, prospects for those in the pool would likely be poor. Data from those 35 states prior to the ACA show that despite charging premiums of nearly 250% more, the solvency of the programs was still questionable. Furthermore, deductibles in those pools reached as high as $25,000 with coverage limits as low as $75,000 [17]. This type of coverage was unaffordable for many with preexisting conditions, was generally inadequate coverage, and cost the system more overall. There is concern that reverting to high-risk pools would bring back many of these consequences.

Interstate Health Insurance Marketplace

One of the consequences of the health insurance marketplace has been heavy consolidation in the industry that has left consumers with few firms to choose from. Fundamental economic theory indicates that as the number of firms decreases, prices for their products increase. Some portion of currently high premium rates may, in fact, be due to a lack of firm-level competition in insurance marketplaces. Indeed, this year 32% of US counties have been left with just one insurer on the exchanges [18]. Republican health plans argue that allowing insurance plans to be purchased across state and county lines would increase competition and drive down premium costs. The danger with such a proposal would be the inevitable race for insurers to establish themselves in the least regulated state. This would lead to a complete loss in states' ability to effectively regulate the insurance market, and coverage quality would likely suffer.

Tort Reform

One criticism of the ACA was that, contrary to expectations, it did not directly address medical malpractice reform. Most Republican health reform alternatives include provisions to address malpractice tort reform. Tort reform proposals are discussed in the Medical Malpractice section at the end of this chapter.

Medicare

Bringing Care to the Elderly: A History

The roots of Medicare lie within Franklin D. Roosevelt's post-Depression New Deal. In the original iterations of the Social Security Act (SSA), which was officially signed in 1935, there were provisions including a national federal health insurance program. Opposition from physician groups led to its removal before the SSA was signed into law. That opposition again prevented similar legislation from being passed under President Harry Truman in the 1940s. As an homage, President Lyndon B. Johnson flew to Truman's hometown of Independence, Missouri, in 1965 to sign the bill enacting Medicare into law as an amendment to the SSA. This insured the nation's elderly, defined by the law as those older than the age of 65.

A number of other groups have been extended Medicare coverage since its passage. In 1972, individuals with permanent disabilities along with those with end-stage renal disease were added to the program. In 2001, those suffering from amyotrophic lateral sclerosis were covered as well. Today, roughly 55 million people receive insurance coverage through the Medicare program, 84% of whom are elderly [19].

The Program

As it stands today, the Medicare program consists of four parts, aptly named Part A, Part B, Part C, and Part D. Medicare Part A insures services performed during a hospital stay, save for "physician services." While there is no premium for elderly patients, they are responsible for a deductible before the Part A coverage kicks in, which is currently $1316. The plan will then cover 60 days of inpatient stay, with an additional 30 days available for a copay currently priced at $322 per day. There are also 60 "lifetime reserve" days available throughout the patient's lifetime that are available at a copay of currently $658 per day. Beyond those days, the patient bears all costs. Part A also covers skilled nursing facility costs, if there is a specific medical need, for 20 days. An additional 80 days are available for a current copay of $164.50 per day. Finally, the Social Security Act was amended in 1982 for Medicare Part A to cover hospice care for patients with a life expectancy of 6 months or less.

Medicare Part B covers outpatient services, as well as inpatient physician services. This includes physical therapy, outpatient surgery, and drugs that must be administered by a physician, such as chemotherapy or immunizations. It also covers some Durable Medical Equipment, including walkers and prosthetics. Part B is a voluntary addition to the Medicare plan, with a premium of around $100 deducted from the individual's social security check, which most elderly beneficiaries elect to do.

In terms of reimbursements from Part B, physicians have a choice on how they prefer to be paid by Medicare. They can either "participate" or "not participate" in the Medicare assignment, which refers to the allowable fees that Medicare sets for services. If the physician participates, he or she will set fees at that level as payment in full. Medicare will then reimburse the doctor directly for 80% of the fee amount, and the remaining 20% is borne by the patient as coinsurance. If the physician does not participate, he or she can charge a fee higher than the allowable fees, up to a maximum of 115% the allowable amount. The patient then becomes responsible for the full amount of the physician's fee, and Medicare will instead reimburse the *patient* 80% of the allowable fee amount. Approximately, 50% of physicians choose not to accept the Medicare assignment, perhaps motivated by the fact that Medicare reimburses on average 2/3 of what private insurance does [20].

Medicare Part C encompasses the Medicare Advantage Plans, which provide private insurance in a managed care model (explained further later in this chapter). The component was initiated with the passage of the Balanced Budget Act of 1997 to address the increasing cost of Medicare. The plans are available to beneficiaries who are already enrolled in Parts A and B, but through managed care mechanisms often realize cost savings that are partly passed on to the consumer. This is often achieved, though, by making available a smaller network of physicians covered to treat the beneficiary.

In 2006, Medicare Part D was implemented to provide beneficiaries insurance against prescription drug costs. However, citing rapidly increasing drug costs, politicians were concerned with letting the government bear the entire financing of the Part D plan. This led the prescription drug component of Medicare to be funded by both the public, through taxes, and privately by beneficiaries, through deductibles and coinsurance. As a result, Medicare Part D plans are offered by private insurance companies, the argument being that choices among the amount and type of coverage offered creates competition to control some of the costs.

Other than a deductible, which is currently capped at $400, beneficiaries of Medicare Part D are responsible for coinsurance. Part D plans will pay 25% of annual drug costs for their beneficiaries up to $3700 annually, with the beneficiary responsible for the remaining 75%. Once annual prescription drug costs exceed $4950, however, the beneficiary becomes eligible for *catastrophic coverage*. This allows him or her to pay very small copays for prescriptions, with the plan covering nearly all of the cost. Between $3700 and $4950, however, there is a clear coverage gap, known as the "donut hole." Figure 11.4 shows what the donut hole looked like prior to the ACA in 2010. The ACA did include provisions to shrink this coverage gap, and today Medicare Part D will cover 60% of the cost of brand name drugs and 49% of the cost of generic drugs within the coverage gap.

Finally, as noted above, there is still a great deal of medical expenditure that Medicare beneficiaries are responsible for. For this reason, many elect to purchase additional insurance coverage for these expenses, commonly known as Medigap or Medicare supplementary insurance. Approximately, 20% of Medicare beneficiaries choose to purchase these plans [22].

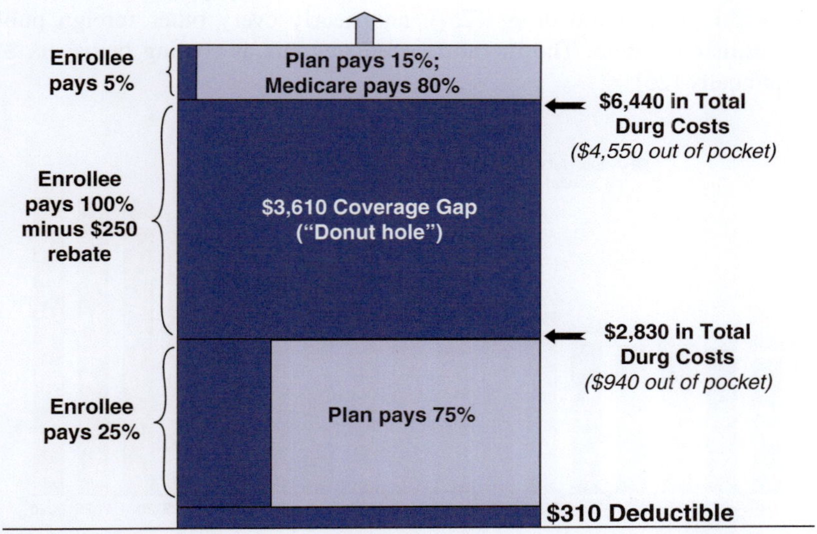

SOURCE: Kaiser Family Foundation illustration of standard Medicare drug benefit for 2010 (standard benefit parameter update from Centers for Medicare & Medicaid Services, April 2009).

Fig. 11.4 Standard Medicare prescription drug benefit, 2010 [21]. The "Donut hole" represents the range in which a beneficiary's drug costs are too high to qualify for plan benefits, but too low to qualify for Medicare catastrophic coverage. Thus, the beneficiary bears 100% of the drug costs. (Reprinted from Ref. [21])

Current Debate

Much of the debate surrounding Medicare is focused on the toll it takes on national expenditures. The program costs over $500 billion annually, representing 14.6% of federal outlays, and is projected to double by 2026 (Fig. 11.5). As the Baby Boomer generation continues to age and the relative proportion of working adults shrinks, the program's sustainability has been called into question. There have been a number of proposals to attempt to curb the rising costs of Medicare. The most common focuses on increasing the age of eligibility for the program in order to shrink the pool that the government supports. Others suggest increasing the amount of cost that beneficiaries must share, through increased premiums, deductibles, or coinsurance rates. Others still propose increasing the Medicare tax that funds the program; the Congressional Budget Office estimates that a 1% increase in the Medicare payroll tax would bring in additional revenues of $823 billion by 2026 and fund the program for decades [23].

Another issue of debate regarding Medicare is centered on the Part D component. The legislation that implemented it prevents the Centers for Medicare & Medicaid Services (CMS) from negotiating drug prices with pharmaceutical companies, despite the fact that it is by far the largest volume purchaser. This is contrary to the abilities granted to other domestic health insurance programs, such as the Veterans Affairs system (who traditionally pays 40–60% less than Medicare for prescription drugs [25]), and nearly every other foreign public health insurance system. The literature estimates this as costing taxpayers $50 billion annually [26].

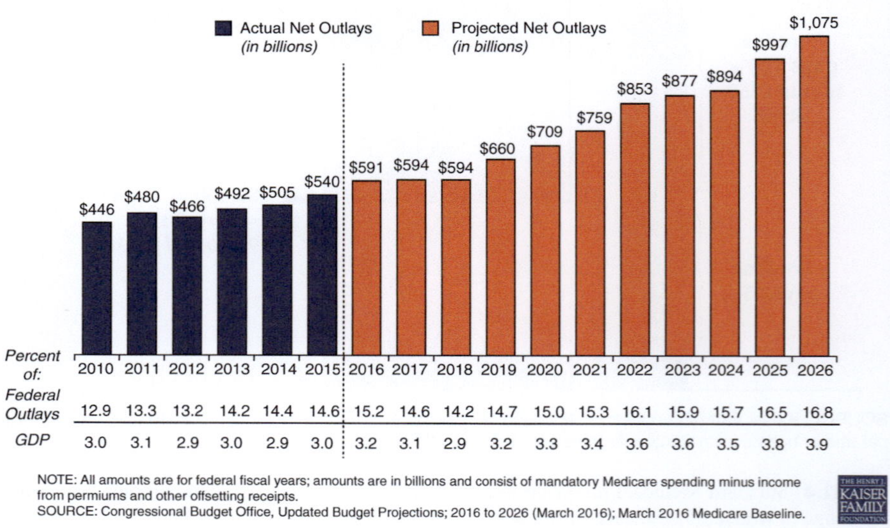

Fig. 11.5 Actual and projected net Medicare spending, 2010–2026 [24]. (Reprinted from Cubanski and Neuman [24])

There is also discussion around how Medicare calculates reimbursement to physicians. Prior to 1992, Medicare Part B would simply reimburse 80% of what it referred to as the "usual, reasonable, and customary charge (UCR)," which was the weighted average of fees that other physicians in the community were charging for the same service. Citing concern that the UCRs were somewhat arbitrary, Congress attempted to design a fee schedule that was more directly related to the resources used to render services. This led to the creation of the Resource-Based Relative Value Scale (RBRVS), which ties fees to resources used, measured by Relative Value Units (RVUs). Controversy around this system has centered on primarily two issues. First, the system tends to favor procedure-based specialties over primary care. This was especially true when the program was initially implemented, as it had reimbursed procedural RVUs more than those involved in evaluation and management [25]. Since then, CMS has increased management and evaluation reimbursements and decreased procedural reimbursements. Second, the RBRVS system has effectively given Medicare, the largest insurer in the nation, the unilateral ability to set reimbursement rates, with many commercial insurers now using Medicare fee schedules as a reference point for contract negotiation. This has reduced physician reimbursement and has been seen as a substantial shift in power over physician compensation.

Medicaid

To insure the nation's poor, Medicaid was established at the same time as Medicare in 1965 with a similar amendment to the SSA. Unlike Medicare, however, the administration of Medicaid has been delegated to the states, each of which does so differently. The federal government instead issues per capita, income-adjusted federal funds to aid in the financing of the programs. On average, the federal government subsidizes 60% of the cost, with the states covering the remainder [27]. The subsidies increase as per capita income in a state decreases. Today, the program covers 74 million Americans, making it the largest insurance program by number of beneficiaries [28].

The Beneficiaries

Medicaid eligibility is dependent upon income levels. The federal poverty level (FPL), defined as the basic level of income, tracks the consumer price index (CPI), a measure of inflation. Today, it sits at $11,880 for an individual, plus $4140 for each dependent. Thus, for a family of 4, the FPL is $24,300. There are certain mandatory groups, including children, adults living with children, and pregnant women, that are to be covered once their incomes fall below 133% of the FPL ($15,800 for an individual and $32,319 for a family of 4). States can also cover these groups, along with a number of "optional groups," under the federal subsidy guidelines up to a maximum of 250% of the FPL ($29,700 for an individual and $60,750 for a family of 4). Childless adults are an optional group that, prior to the ACA, was almost never covered. The ACA specifically targeted this group in its provision to expand Medicaid, which will be discussed further in this section. Prior to the ACA, 49 million individuals were enrolled in the Medicaid program (Fig. 11.6).

The ACA's Bid to Expand Medicaid

Passage of the ACA included a provision that pushed expansion of state Medicaid programs to all individuals, including childless adults, and increased the floor from 133% to 138% of the FPL. This was the reason why subsidies on the exchanges were only offered beginning at 133% of the FPL, rather than making them available to the poor. To account for the costs of expansion, the federal government would increase its federal subsidies to states to manage 100% of the cost, phasing down to a steady level of 90% by 2020.

However, this provision of the ACA mandated that states expand their Medicaid programs or lose the federal funding already allotted to their programs. This became controversial, because although every state did implement a Medicaid program, the original language of the amendment to the SSA technically indicated Medicaid as a *voluntary* program. This debate was included in the *National Federation of Independent Businesses v. Sebelius* hearing that reached the Supreme Court. Though the Supreme Court upheld the individual mandate portion of that case, they ruled that Congress had

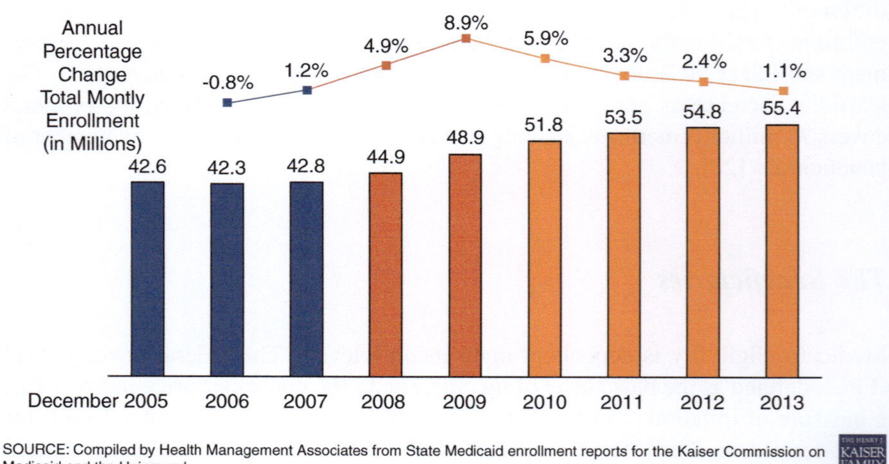

Fig. 11.6 Annual change in total Medicaid enrollment, December 2005–December 2013 [29]. (Reprinted from Snyder and Rudowitz [29])

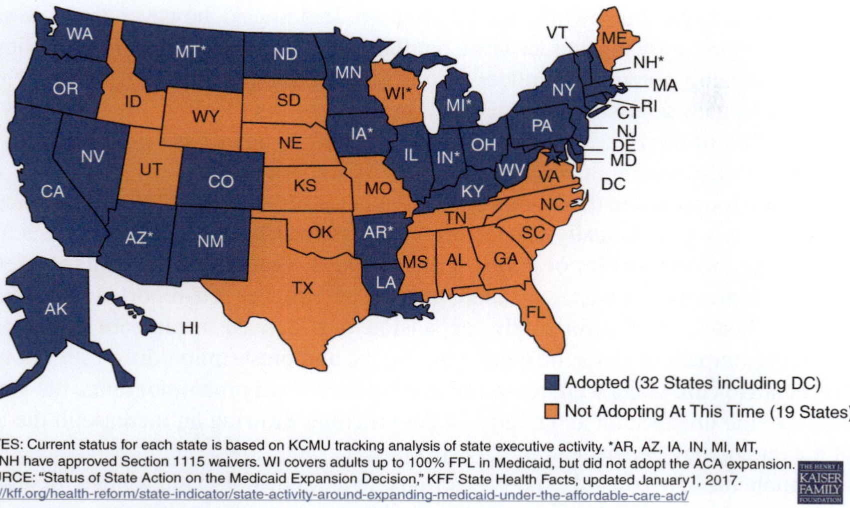

Fig. 11.7 Status of state Medicaid expansion decisions, 2017 [31]. *AR, AZ, IA, IN, MI, MT, and NH have applied Section 1115 Waivers that allow changes in eligibility, benefit, cost sharing, and/or provider payment requirements. Though Wisconsin has not adopted the ACA's Medicaid expansion, it has chosen to cover adults up to 100% (rather than 138%) of the FPL. (Reprinted from Ref. [31])

exceeded its spending power in coercing states to expand their Medicaid programs without funding it in its entirety. Thus, Medicaid expansion became an optional, state-decided provision of the ACA, and to this day only 32 states and the District of Columbia have chosen to expand (Fig. 11.7). Wisconsin, though not officially expanding its program, is the only other state to extend Medicaid coverage to childless adults, albeit only for those below 100% of the FPL rather than 138% [30].

In addition to expanding the Medicaid program, the ACA created the CMS Innovation Center within CMS. This organization was given funding to distribute grants to state governments and private entities to experiment with novel healthcare delivery systems. To date, the Innovation Center has funded 39 models, and the Congressional Budget Office forecasts it saving the federal government $34 billion in healthcare expenditures by 2026 [32]. It is through the Innovation Center that the Comprehensive Care for Joint Replacement program was conceived, which now reimburses joint replacement surgery from Medicare on a strictly bundled payment structure in certain geographies (explained in detail later in this chapter).

Oregon's Rare Experiment

Much of the argument in support of Medicaid expansion, and in support of increased access to health insurance in general, rests on the assumption that insured individuals should be more likely to use cheaper, more preventative health measures rather than costlier emergency care. In 2008, just prior to passage of the ACA, Oregon took steps to expand its own Medicaid program. In doing so, however, the state saw a unique opportunity to conduct a rare randomized-controlled trial in health policy – by randomizing potential enrollees into a lottery that determined whether or not they would gain access to the program. Though it set its threshold for eligibility at below 100% of the FPL, rather than the ACA's 138%, states have used the study in evaluating the decision of whether or not to expand Medicaid.

Oregon found that in the 2 years that it conducted the trial, enrollment in Medicaid did not have any statistically significant impact on measures of health status such as blood pressure or markers of diabetes management, except for reducing the prevalence of depression. It was associated, though, with higher self-reported mental and physical health. Not surprisingly, expansion did increase healthcare utilization, including outpatient visits, hospital admissions, and prescription drug use. Though preventative care visits were more utilized, such as yearly mammograms, the study did have the unexpected and controversial outcome showing an increase in the use of the emergency department by 20% [33].

Opponents of Medicaid expansion often cite this study as evidence that Medicaid does not achieve what it is intended to, and could increase healthcare costs in the long run. Proponents respond with a number of limitations regarding the trial. Generalizability of the results beyond one state has been called into question, as has the potential effect of using a 138% threshold instead of 100%. But perhaps most debatable is the 2-year timeline of the study, which proponents of Medicaid expansion argue is simply not long enough to determine the long-term behavioral changes that insurance coverage is supposed to drive.

Effects of Expanding

States that chose to expand their Medicaid programs expectedly saw increased spending to implement the expansion. In the 29 states that had expanded Medicaid by 2015, spending increased by 17.7% on average, compared to a 6.1% increase in nonexpansion states. Also not surprisingly, expansion states saw increases in insurance coverage of their populace. In those same 29 states, enrollment in Medicaid increased 18% on average, compared to 5.1% in the remaining states [34]. Whether or not this increased enrollment leads to better "access to care" is still in question. Some studies have shown significant increases in access to a personal physician or to necessary medications in expansion states [35]. The literature, however, does not show a consensus that Medicaid expansion does necessarily improve measures of healthcare accessibility [36].

It does appear that expansion of Medicaid increases healthcare utilization, at least as measured by overnight hospitalizations and physician visits. There has also been improvement in the rates of diagnosis of chronic diseases, such as diabetes and hypercholesterolemia, among the Medicaid population. Interestingly, there has not been an increase in emergency department utilization as the Oregon study may have suggested [36]. Economically, results have been positive. Expansion states have actually realized revenue gains, budget savings, and overall economic growth [37].

The Managed Care Model

Managed care is an umbrella term that refers to a number of techniques, employed by Managed Care Organizations (MCOs), to control the process of healthcare delivery, from financing to providing, in order to reduce cost. MCOs act both as insurers, by negotiating and collecting premiums from its members, and as providers of care, by arranging for the patient to be seen by more limited networks of physicians. The model of managed care relies on the concept that choice is costly, and that one way to manage cost is to limit choice.

MCOs further innovated by shifting reimbursement structures away from the fee-for-service (FFS) model, attempting to tie financial incentives toward outcomes. This led to a number of different approaches to attempt to "pay-for-performance (PFP)." The argument for financially rewarding favorable outcome metrics is twofold. First, the traditional FFS model has the unfortunate incentive that rewards additional care, regardless of necessity. While the question of whether this actually incentivizes physicians to overutilize services is up for debate, it certainly does not penalize it. Second, tying incentives to clinically desirable outcome measures theoretically has the potential to improve quality of care overall.

The Health Maintenance Organization

Where we left off in the first section of this chapter, managed care was slowly beginning to take center stage in healthcare administration, namely, in the form of the Health Maintenance Organization (HMO). Of all MCOs, the HMO is the most limiting in terms of choice. Like other MCOs, there is a defined network of physicians that the organization has negotiated with to provide care. This network can come in a number of different ways. From most restrictive to least, the network can be literally employed by the HMO, such as with Kaiser Permanente's model, the HMO can contract with a single extant group practice or hospital, or the HMO can contract individually with a number of groups or solo practices. The Independent Practice Association model, which really is just a subtype of the HMO, chooses an intermediary organization to contract out physicians on its behalf. Whatever the defined network, the patient must be treated by a physician that is "in" the network under the plan.

Part of the HMO's strategy is heavy utilization of the "gatekeeper" concept. This setup puts the primary care physician in charge of coordinating all of the health services that a patient needs. All specialty care requires referral from the gatekeeper primary care physician in an attempt to reduce overutilization of more costly care.

It also works to emphasize more preventative care measures through better utilizing the primary care physician. An emphasis on preventative care became a technique to try to reduce long-term costs.

Physician reimbursement in the HMO follows a capitation model. Capitation pays physicians a set annual fee per patient that the physician is responsible for caring for. This is a PFP design in which the performance metric is cost. If the physician is able to care for the patient utilizing less in financial resources than the fee he or she receives, he or she makes a profit. If, however, the costs of care rise above the fee paid, the physician eats the loss.

The Preferred Provider Organization

The HMO's strict restrictiveness with regard to its network of physicians led it to fall out of favor in the 1990s. Patients laid blame onto their HMOs when they could not see the physician they wanted to or when treatments were denied, leading to a feeling that administrators were getting too involved in actual patient care. This led to the development of the Preferred Provider Organization (PPO), which implemented an additional layer of choice onto the HMO model. PPOs allow their members to visit "out-of-network" physicians, but at a higher copayment fee than those who were "in-network." They also less frequently utilize the gatekeeper structure.

Rather than work off of capitation, the PPO model usually negotiates discounts from its in-network physicians. These discounts generally range between 25% and 35% [38].

The Accountable Care Organization

The ACA's answer to managed care was the Accountable Care Organization (ACO), which forms a sort of hybrid between the HMO and PPO. Though there is an ACO "network," members are not limited to seeking care from within the network. Any and all costs incurred by the patient, in or out of network, though, are "accountable" to the ACO. These organizations emphasize care quality metrics and seek to provide integrated care that encompasses all of the patient's needs. ACOs were given an official designation under the ACA, provided they meet a set of requirements, including having a minimum patient base of 5000 that it manages for at least 3 years. The organizations make extensive use of PFP reimbursement structures to attempt to incentivize both quality and cost efficiency. Many ACOs continue to employ a modified FFS in which providers share cost savings with the ACO. More controversial is the bundled payment reimbursement structure, which has been increasing in popularity and recently became Medicare's standard reimbursement model for joint replacement surgery.

Bundled Payments

Bundled payments have been proposed as a middle ground between the traditional FFS reimbursement structure and the capitation payment model of the HMO years. It retains the concept of flat fees that characterized capitation reimbursements in order to share cost savings with providers, but does so on a procedural, rather than per patient, basis. The idea stems from the Diagnosis-Related Group (DRG) system that Medicare began employing in the 1980s to reimburse physicians flat fees for treatment of a "diagnosis" that a patient received. It, too, was designed to shift cost risks over to providers in an attempt to incentivize cost reduction. However, critics claimed that it might have inadvertently incentivized providers to seek earlier discharge for their patients. In responding to that criticism, bundled payments combine both the inpatient treatment and the posthospital outcomes together in an "episode of care." This translates to costs incurred for a defined period after discharge still being covered by the fixed umbrella payment for that episode. Analysis of the potential savings of bundled payment initiatives has been promising – a study of the 17 most costly procedures benchmarked to costs of the 50th percentile shows potential savings of $4.7 billion annually [39].

In 2006, a bundled payment package was introduced by Geisinger Health System targeted at coronary artery bypass surgery. ProvenCare established a fixed payment to coronary surgeons for preoperative care, operative care, and 90 days of postoperative care. The program led to decreased lengths of stay, higher rates of discharge to home, and lower readmissions [40]. In 2011, Medicare announced a pilot bundled payment program dubbed the Bundled Payments for Care Improvement (BPCI) initiative. It is a voluntary program that uses bundled payments to reimburse 48 different DRGs that providers can choose from, spanning from myocardial infarction to joint replacement surgery to sepsis. The program is currently in its second phase, in which nearly 1400 groups have chosen to participate for at least one of the episodes [41].

While the full results of the pilot have not yet been released, preliminary data show mixed results. So far, most of the clinical episodes have *not* shown reduced costs since the implementation of BPCI. Orthopedic surgery episodes, composed primarily of hip and knee arthroplasties, however, have achieved positive results. Specifically for orthopedic episodes, 89% of groups saw declines in payments, and on average, total standardized allowed payments declined by $2137 (Fig. 11.8). The decline was attributed to changes in post-acute care during the 90-day postoperative episode duration. The percentage of patients discharged to home increased from 36% to 43%, and average length of stay at a skilled nursing facility was 1.3 days shorter for the BPCI episodes. For nearly all quality metrics, however, including readmission rates, emergency room visits, and mortality rates, there has been no statistically significant difference for BPCI episodes [42].

Within the last year, the same CMS Innovation Center that implemented the BPCI designed and executed the Comprehensive Care for Joint Replacement (CJR) model. This time an involuntary program, CJR, altered Medicare reimbursement

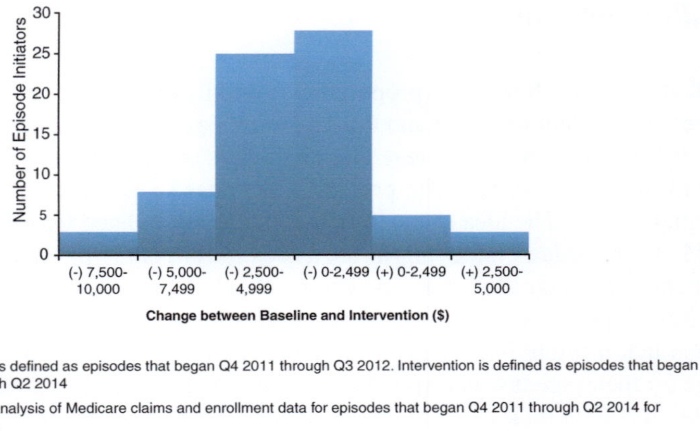

Fig. 11.8 Distribution of the average change in total standardized allowed payments for orthopedic surgery episodes after initiation of bundled payments [43]. These payments represent payments to Medicare Parts A and B services. The timeline of payments extends from the anchor hospitalization to 90 days postoperatively. (Reprinted from Dummit et al. [43])

policy for DRGs 469 and 470 (knee and hip arthroplasties) to be done as bundled payments. The episode of care has been defined as the duration from admission to the hospital up until 90 days after discharge. The model applies on a mandatory basis to approximately 800 hospitals in 67 defined geographic regions across the country. The impact of this change is uncertain, but opponents are concerned about the level of risk being shifted onto providers with these changes. Further, CMS denied a request to adjust the bundled payments based on the risk pool of patients treated, leading to additional controversy. What is certain is that the movement toward pay-for-performance will continue a focus of healthcare reform in the modern day, and orthopedic surgery has become a primary target on which to trial these techniques.

Medical Malpractice

By the age 65, 88.5% of medical doctors and 98.4% of surgeons will face a malpractice claim [44]. Medical malpractice is a type of *tort*, or civil wrongdoing (in contrast to a criminal one). Tort law is designed to protect individuals from wrongdoing that is not necessarily a crime. Malpractice claims allow the courts to financially rectify harms suffered by patients. Tort reform with respect to medical malpractice has also entered into health policy reform discussions. Advocates of tort reform argue that lax tort laws both drive up the costs of malpractice insurance and lead to the practice of defensive medicine – a costly consequence whereby physicians order sometimes unnecessary tests in order to reduce the likelihood of missing something that could lead to a lawsuit down the road. In addition, it has been noted that the current tort system does not deter medical errors or encourage adverse event reporting, and that injured patients receive less than half of the total expenditure on malpractice insurance [45]. Conservative estimates of the costs of defensive medicine are about $50 billion annually [46]. While this only represents 2% of total healthcare expenditures, malpractice premium shocks of up to 30% at the turn of the millennium led to serious pushes for tort reform [47].

Tort Reform Proposals

Malpractice Caps

A commonly employed tort reform technique is to limit the potentially high payouts of malpractice claims. Less costly claims make it less risky to insure those claims, and in theory should reduce malpractice insurance premiums. When employed, caps on malpractice suit payouts are placed on the "noneconomic damages" of the claim. When a malpractice suit is filed, there are two categories of damages that a plaintiff can lay claim to economic and noneconomic damages. Economic damages refer to those harms that can be directly tied to monetary losses, such as medical bills, lost income/earning capacity, and household services required. They are often relatively easy to quantify in the lawsuit. Noneconomic damages, on the other hand, refer to everything else. States vary in their definitions of noneconomic damages, but they often include compensation for things like pain and suffering, humiliation, or reputational damage. Though much harder to quantify than economic damages, when awarded they are often significantly costlier.

Currently, there are 32 states that employ caps on noneconomic damages for malpractice suits, ranging from $250,000 up to $2,250,000 (Fig. 11.9). These caps do appear to at least achieve the goal of reduced malpractice insurance premiums; in comparing states with caps to states without caps, premium increases in 2001 were 72% lower [48]. Whether or not these caps have any effect on defensive medicine practices is inconclusive in the literature [49].

Tribunal Panels

An issue that has been raised in cases of medical malpractice is that, stemming from the relative complexity of medical decision-making, a lay jury or judge might not be qualified to render a verdict. To address this, some have advocated for the use of professional tribunals in malpractice suits. This would modify the way in which malpractice cases are ruled upon, using instead a panel of judges with specific medical expertise that would enable them to appropriately assess the case. This was experimented with in Massachusetts, who currently offers Medical

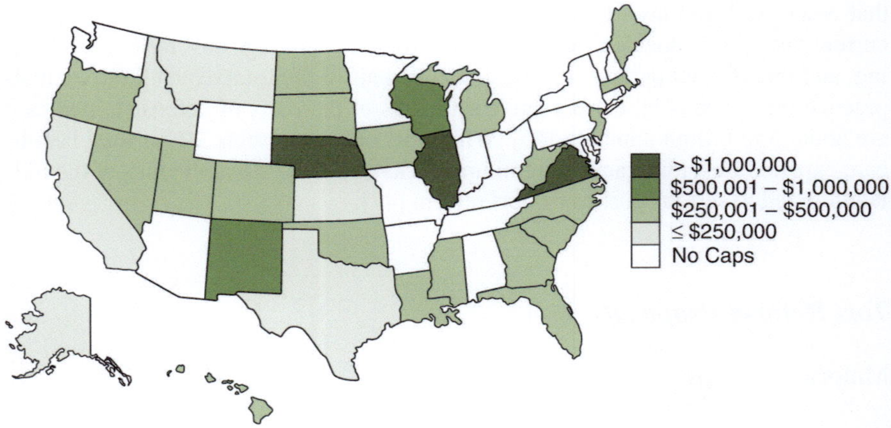

Fig. 11.9 State caps on noneconomic damages for malpractice suits, 2016

Malpractice Tribunals at the request of the defendant. An early evaluation of the program showed that roughly two-thirds of cases presented before the tribunal are thrown out as merely an "unfortunate medical result" [50].

Disclosure-and-Offer Programs

Though not a formal legal reform, disclosure-and-offer programs are an interesting way for providers to take charge in reducing litigation on their own. These are programs, often implemented at large hospitals or groups, in which physicians immediately disclose adverse events to patients and offer compensation if appropriate. While the patient retains the right to file a lawsuit, these programs have been shown to significantly reduce the chance of that happening. The University of Michigan found that after implementing a disclosure-and-offer program, the rate of lawsuits fell from 2.3 per 100,000 physicians to just 0.75. The duration of the process became shorter as well, and costs decreased overall [51]. Disclosure-and-offer programs are also interesting in that they often involve an apology when errors occur.

Apologies have been shown in the literature to reduce the number of lawsuits filed by 50–65%, and to substantially reduce the financial payouts from those suits [52]. There is some controversy regarding apologizing during a disclosure of medical error, however, considering state environments regarding their legal definitions. States differ on whether or not they permit apologies, which could be as simple as an expression of sympathy, or disclosures to be admissible in court as admissions of fault. Currently, 34 states have "apology laws" preventing physician apologies from being used as evidence of liability. Nine states have similar laws for any kind of disclosure of medical error (Table 11.2) [53]. Lawyers, therefore, have given conflicting advice on the subject of whether or not to include an apology with a disclosure of medical error from a medicolegal standpoint. Apology laws have been

Table 11.2 Overview of state apology and disclosure laws

Both disclosure and apology laws	Apology laws only	Disclosure laws only	Neither
California	Arizona	Nevada	Alabama
Florida	Colorado	New Jersey	Alaska
Oregon	Connecticut	Pennsylvania	Arkansas
Tennessee	Delaware		Illinois
Vermont	Georgia		Kansas
Washington	Hawaii		Kentucky
	Idaho		Michigan
	Indiana		Minnesota
	Iowa		Mississippi
	Louisiana		New Mexico
	Maine		New York
	Maryland		Rhode Island
	Massachusetts		Wisconsin
	Missouri		
	Montana		
	Nebraska		
	New Hampshire		
	North Carolina		
	North Dakota		
	Ohio		
	Oklahoma		
	South Carolina		
	South Dakota		
	Texas		
	Utah		
	Virginia		
	West Virginia		
	Wyoming		

shown to be associated with reduced average settlement payments as well as fewer cases involving minor injury, and as such have developed their own discussion in the tort reform debate [54].

Safe Harbor Laws

Another proposed reform to the malpractice system is the implementation of a safe harbor to protect from liability physicians who have adhered to an evidence-based practice guideline. Proponents argue that if a physician has followed such a guideline, such a case should be and would be ruled in his or her favor anyways. A safe harbor would protect from frivolous lawsuits, as well as outlier cases in which physicians are held liable for errors that result from following accepted practice guidelines. Some physicians are wary, however, of conceding that much power over the nuances of the practice of medicine to guidelines, and of the ambiguity of what is considered "scientific evidence."

References

1. Musgrove P, Creese A, Preker A, Baeza C, Anell A, Prentic T. Health systems: improving performance. Geneva: The World Health Organization; 2000. Final Report.
2. Shi L, Singh D. Historical overview of US health care delivery. In: Shi L, Singh D, editors. Essentials of the US healthcare system. Sudbury: Jones and Bartlett Publishers; 2005. p. 45–69.
3. Shi L, Singh D. Essentials of the US healthcare system. Sudbury: Jones and Bartlett Publishers; 2005. Figure 9.1, Average annual rates of increase in National Health Expenditures (NHE), Gross Domestic Product (GDP), and Consumer Price Index (CPI); 1966–1971. p. 224.
4. Barnett JC, Vornovitsky MS. Health insurance coverage in the United States: 2015. Washington DC: U.S. Government Printing Office; 2016. Report No.: P60–257 (RV).
5. Medicaid and Medicare at 50: trends and challenges [PowerPoint Presentation]. Menlo Park: The Henry J. Kaiser Family Foundation; 2015 [cited 2017 Mar 3]. [Figure], Medicaid and Medicare Together Provide Health Insurance Coverage for More than 3 in 10 Americans; Slide 1. Available from: http://kff.org/slideshow/medicaid-and-medicare-at-50-trends-and-challenges/.
6. Skinner JS, Staiger DO, Fisher ES. Is technological change in medicine always worth it? The case of acute myocardial infarction. Health Aff (Millwood). 2006;25(2):w34–47. Exhibit 4, Change In Survival And Change In Medicare Spending, By Hospital Referral Region (HRR), 1986–2002; p. W39.
7. Global Health Observatory Data [Internet]. Geneva (Switzerland): The World Health Organization. c2016 – [cited 2017 Feb 10]. Available from: http://www.who.int/gho/database/en/.
8. Brasfield J. health care reform: the dream deferred. In: Brasfield J, editor. Health policy: the decade ahead. Boulder: Lynne Rienner Publishers, Inc.; 2011. p. 165–202.
9. Kane J. Health costs: how the U.S. compares with other countries. 2012 Oct 22 [cited 2017 Feb 13]. In: PBS Newshour: The Rundown [Internet]. [Figure], US spends two-and-a-half times the OECD average; [about 1 screen]. Available from: http://www.pbs.org/newshour/rundown/health-costs-how-the-us-compares-with-other-countries/Kirchhoff SM.
10. Medical loss ratio requirements under the patient protection and Affordable Care Act (ACA): issues for congress. Congressional Research Service. 2014 Aug 26.
11. Overview of the uninsured in the United States: a summary of the 2011 current population survey. Washington DC: Office of the Assistant Secretary for Planning and Evaluation; 2011 Sep 13. Figure 4, Profile of the Uninsured vs. Total Population by Age, 2010; p. 4.
12. Cantor JC, Monheit AC, DeLia D, Lloyd K. Early impact of the Affordable Care Act on health insurance coverage of young adults. Health Serv Res. 2012;47(5):1773–90.
13. Mathur A, Slavov SN, Strain MR. Has the Affordable Care Act increased part-time employment? Appl Econ Lett. 2015;23(3):222–225.
14. Saltzman E, Eibner C. Donald Trump's health care reform proposals: anticipated effects on insurance coverage, Out-of-Pocket Costs, and the Federal Deficit. Washington DC: The Commonwealth Fund; 2016.
15. Gorenstein D. With a high deductible, even a doctor can shortchange his health. Kaiser Health News. 2017 Feb 8.
16. Medicaid Managed Care Trends and Snapshots: 2000–2013. Washington DC: Centers for Medicare & Medicaid Services; 2013.

17. Comprehensive health insurance for high-risk individuals: a state-by-state analysis. Denver: National Association of State Comprehensive Health Insurance Plans; 2012/2013.
18. Armour S, Mathews AW. New rule aims to calm insurers. Wall Street J. 2017;Sect. A:5 (col. 3).
19. 2015 CMS Statistics [Internet]. Washington (DC): Centers for Medicare & Medicaid Services. c2015 – [cited 2017 Feb 11]. Available from: https://www.cms.gov/Research-Statistics-Data-and-Systems/Statistics-Trends-and-Reports/CMS-Statistics-Reference-Booklet/Downloads/2015CMSStatistics.pdf#page=12.
20. Barr DA. Medicare. In: Barr DA, editor. U.S. health policy: The Organization, financing, and delivery of health care in America. San Francisco: Pearson; 2002. p. 89–107.
21. Medicare: a primer. Menlo Park: The Henry J. Kaiser Family Foundation. 2010. Standard medicare prescription drug benefit; 2010. p. 7.
22. An overview of medicare. Menlo Park: The Henry J. Kaiser Family Foundation; 2016.
23. Options for reducing the deficit: 2017 to 2026. Washington: The Congressional Budget Office. 2016 Dec 8. Nonpartisan Analysis.
24. Cubanski J, Neuman T. The facts on medicare spending and financing. Menlo Park: The Henry J. Kaiser Family Foundation. 2016 . Figure 4, Actual and Projected Net Medicare Spending, 2010–2026; p. 3.
25. Duston PS. Taking care of the elderly. In: Duston PS, editor. Analyzing form, function, and financing of the U.S. Health Care System. Boca Raton: Taylor & Francis Group, LLC; 2016. p. 319–34.
26. Frakt AB, Pizer SD, Feldman R. Should medicare adopt the Veterans Health Administration formulary? Health Econ. 2012 May;21(5):485–95.
27. Barr DA. Medicaid. In: Barr DA, editor. U.S. health policy: The Organization, financing, and delivery of health care in America. San Francisco: Pearson; 2002. p. 108–25.
28. Total monthly medicaid and CHIP enrollment [Internet]. Menlo Park: The Henry J. Kaiser Family Foundation. c2016 – [cited 2017 Feb 12]. Available from: http://kff.org/health-reform/state-indicator/total-monthly-medicaid-and-chip-enrollment/?currentTimeframe=0.
29. Snyder L, Rudowitz R. Medicaid Enrollment: December 2013 Data Snapshot. Menlo Park: The Henry J. Kaiser Family Foundation; 2014. Figure 1; Annual Change in Total Medicaid Enrollment, December 2005 to December 2013; p. 1.
30. Where are States today? Medicaid and CHIP eligibility levels for children, pregnant women, and adults. Menlo Park: The Henry J. Kaiser Family Foundation; 2017.
31. Current status of state medicaid expansion decisions [map]. Menlo Park: The Henry J. Kaiser Family Foundation; 2017. Available from: http://kff.org/health-reform/slide/current-status-of-the-medicaid-expansion-decision/.
32. CMS Innovation Center: report to congress. Washington DC: The Centers for Medicare & Medicaid Services; 2016.
33. Baicker K, Taubman SL, Allen HL, Bernstein M, Gruber JH, Newhouse JP, Schneider EC, Wright BJ, Zaslavsky AM, Finkelstein AN. The Oregon experiment--effects of Medicaid on clinical outcomes. N Engl J Med. 2013;368(18):1713–22.
34. Rudowitz R, Snyder L. Medicaid Enrollment & Spending Growth: FY 2015 & 2016. Menlo Park: The Henry J. Kaiser Family Foundation; 2015.
35. Sommers BD, Gunja MZ, Finegold K, Musco T. Changes in self-reported insurance coverage, access to care, and health under the Affordable Care Act. JAMA. 2015;314(4):366–74.
36. Wherry LR, Miller S. Early coverage, access, utilization, and health effects associated with the Affordable Care Act medicaid expansions: a quasi-experimental study. Ann Intern Med. 2016;164(12):795–803.
37. Bachrach D, Howard H. States expanding medicaid see significant budget savings and revenue gains: a presentation to grantmakers in health [PowerPoint Presentation]. Princeton: The Robert Wood Johnson Foundation; 2015.
38. Shi L, Singh D. Managed care and health networks. In: Shi L, Singh D, editors. Essentials of the US healthcare system. Sudbury: Jones and Bartlett Publishers; 2005. p. 197–219.

39. Cutler DM, Ghosh K. The Potential for Cost Savings through Bundled Episode Payments. N Engl J Med. 2012;366:1075–7.
40. Edmonds C, Hallman GL. Cardio vascular care providers. A pioneer in bundled services, shared risk, and single payment. Tex Heart Inst J. 1995;22(1):72.
41. Bundled Payments for Care Improvement (BPCI) Initiative: general information. Washington: The Centers for Medicare & Medicaid Services; 2017.
42. Dummit L, Marrufo G, Marshall J, Tan E, Bradley A, Hall C, et al. CMS bundled payments for care improvement initiative models 2–4: year 2 evaluation & monitoring annual report. The Lewin Group; 2016.
43. Dummit L, Marrufo G, Marshall J, Tan E, Bradley A, Hall C, et al. CMS bundled payments for care improvement initiative models 2–4: year 2 evaluation & monitoring annual report. The Lewin Group. 2016 Aug. Exhibit 53, Distribution of the average change in total standardized allowed payment for part A and B services during the anchor hospitalization and the 90-day PDP for orthopedic surgery episodes, Model 2, intervention relative to baseline; p. 128.
44. Jena AB, Seabury S, Lakdawalla D, Chandra A. Malpractice Risk According to Physician Specialty. N Engl J Med. 2011;365:629–36.
45. Mello MM, Williams CH. Medical malpractice: impact of the crisis and effect of state tort reforms. Princeton: The Robert Wood Johnson Foundation; 2006.
46. Feldman AM. Will we ever see tort reform in the United States? In: Feldman AM, editor. Understanding health care reform. Boca Raton: Taylor & Francis Group; 2012. p. 165–77.
47. Evaluating state approaches to the medical malpractice crisis. Health Policy Monitor 2004; 9(1).
48. Confronting the new health care crisis: improving health care quality and lowering costs by fixing our medical liability system. Washington DC: U.S. Department of Health and Human Services (DHHS), Office of the Assistant Secretary for Planning and Evaluatio; 2002. Available at: http://aspe.hhs.gov/daltcp/reports/litrefm.pdf.
49. Nelson LJ, Morrisey MA, Kilgore ML. Damages Caps in Medical Malpractice Cases. Milbank Q. 2007;85(2):259–86.
50. McLaughlin WH. A look at the Massachusetts malpractice tribunal system. Am J Law Med. 1977;3(2):197–207.
51. Boothman R, Hoyler MM. The University of Michigan's early disclosure and offer program. Bull Am Coll Surg. 2013;98(3):21–5.
52. Sohn DH, Bal BS. Medical malpractice reform: the role of alternative dispute resolution. Clin Orthop Relat Res. 2012;470(5):1370–8.
53. Mastroianni AC, Mello MM, Sommer S, Hardy M, Gallagher TH. The flaws in state 'apology' and 'disclosure' laws dilute their intended impact on malpractice suits. Health Aff (Millwood). 2010;29(9):1611–9.
54. Ho B, Liu E. Does sorry work?. The impact of apology laws on medical malpractice. J Risk Uncert. 2011;43:141.

Part III
Additional Topics

Chapter 12
Surgical Training and Education

Daniel J. Miller and Vasilios (Bill) Moutzouros

Docendo ergo disco: I Teach, Therefore I Learn [1]

Education has been integral to the practice of medicine since its inception. In fact, the word doctor takes its origin from the Latin word *docere,* meaning "to teach." An active role in surgical education provides the orthopedist tremendous opportunity for personal and professional satisfaction. This chapter will provide an introduction to the history, ethics, and practice of modern surgical education with special attention to orthopedic training. We will introduce different strategies that teachers may incorporate to improve the knowledge and skills of orthopedic trainees.

Historical Background

Surgical education has evolved significantly over the past 200 years. In the late nineteenth century, surgeons were entirely self-taught or trained under a single apprentice with minimal, if any regulation [2]. The publishing of the Flexner report in 1910 led to sweeping reforms in medical and surgical education that provided for increased government regulation of medical licensure and training. The Johns Hopkins Hospital, founded in 1889, provided a new framework for formal medical training in a university setting. The Hopkins model of graduated responsibility resulting in eventual autonomy and independent practice remains the prevailing paradigm for medical and surgical education to this day [3].

D. J. Miller
Gillette Children's Specialty Healthcare, St. Paul, MN, USA

V. Moutzouros (✉)
Division of Sports Medicine, Henry Ford Health System, Department of Orthopedic Surgery, Detroit, MI, USA
e-mail: vmoutzo1@hfhs.org

E. C. Makhni et al. (eds.), *Orthopedic Practice Management*,
https://doi.org/10.1007/978-3-319-96938-1_12

The American Board of Orthopedic Surgery (ABOS) was organized in 1935 through the combined efforts of the American Orthopedic Association (AOA), American Academy of Orthopedic Surgeons (AAOS), and the American Medical Association (AMA) [4]. The ABOS established the first formal educational standards for orthopedic surgery in the United States and continues to regulate surgeon certification today [4]. The American Council of Graduate Medical Education (ACGME), founded in 1981, governs accreditation of graduate medical training programs including orthopedic residencies and select fellowships in the United States. ACGME policies have a significant impact on modern-day orthopedic training. In recent years, the ACGME has spearheaded regulations related to work hours, supervision, and breadth of competencies with the ultimate goal of improving patient safety and the trainee experience.

Why Teach?

Educating trainees requires considerable time and effort with few obvious concrete gains. Before reviewing the most effective techniques to teach, it is worth discussing the merits of teaching.

Although education has mainly altruistic goals, it does provide many tangible benefits to the educator. Teaching forces an educator to maintain and expand their own knowledge base, providing an impetus for continued growth and learning. Students and trainees approach new topics and problems with an open mind. As such, their unique perspective may shed new light on a topic to an educator. Trainees can bring knowledge of newly developed ideas or techniques from other subspecialties that may be applicable to the teacher's area of practice.

Many orthopedic educators report personal satisfaction from the connection imparted by teaching. These relationships may bloom in to lifelong professional partnerships. Teaching allows the educator to take pleasure vicariously in the successes and accomplishments of his or her students. In addition to the student-teacher relationship, teaching can also lead to meaningful relationships and partnerships between educators. Experiential teaching also allows for passage of educational experience that cannot be gathered in a book or online module. It allows the teachers to pass on a legacy of experience.

Together with research and patient care, education represents a pillar of the academic medical center. Many surgeons note a professional obligation to teach, as a way of paying back the system that produced them. Education allows an educator to contribute to the greater good of society by ensuring the development of competent and compassionate surgeons. In many ways, the legacy of an educator may have a greater impact compared to their own direct actions.

Challenges to Modern Surgical Education

Teaching, as opposed to mere demonstration or oversight, requires sacrifice on the part of the educator [5]. In particular, effective teaching requires substantial time and energy, provides no financial remuneration, and is associated with decreased clinical productivity. The time, work, and energy dedicated to education are hard to quantify and may be dismissed or undervalued by colleagues or hospital systems. Few means exist to reward outstanding educators for their contributions. On an organizational scale, funding and research support for medical education is weak. In the digital age, new technology and techniques are being developed and disseminated at an unprecedented rate. As a result, surgeons may find themselves needing to devote time and focus to their own clinical skills before worrying about educating others.

Surgical education is also limited by the time constraints on the trainee. Particularly salient to this conversation is the implementation of the ACGME resident duty hour work regulations. These regulations were first incorporated in 2003 with the goal of improving education while decreasing medical errors attributable to sleep deprivation and fatigue [6]. The ACGME work hour regulations have been a source of considerable controversy in orthopedic training [6]. Critics cite concerns regarding continuity of patient care and decreased operative and clinical experience by residents [6]. Data looking at resident education suggests that the work hour regulations do not have a significant detrimental effect on surgical case experience, with some programs reporting increased resident case experience after the new regulations [7, 8]. It should be noted that medical errors have not improved since the inception of the work hour regulations.

The ACGME has been instrumental in reorganizing the Post-Graduate Year-1 (PGY-1) training experience in graduate medical education and orthopedics in recent years. In 2011, ACGME reduced the number of consecutive hours that PGY-1 residents in any field can work in a single shift from 30 to 16 [9]. This led to concern regarding insufficient training time for interns and increased number of patient handoffs. In light of continued research and feedback, the ACGME is expected to increase the number of allowable consecutive hours for interns to 24 in the coming future.

Regardless of the effect of ACGME regulations, time in residency training is limited in relation to the ever-expanding orthopedic knowledge base and technical arsenal. Emphasis should be placed at maximizing learning from all available opportunities that exist in the workplace [10].

Although education has been recognized as an integral part of the academic training model, little attention has been given to teaching as a skill in its own right. While licensing committees and board certification promote and maintain standardizations for practice, no such board certifies or monitors educators. For the history of medicine, physicians have been given little to no training on how to be an effective educator. Apart from the AAOS orthopedic educators course, few resources exist to help orthopedic surgeons to improve their teaching skills. All too often, great physicians and great surgeons are assumed to be great educators. While knowledge and skill are prerequisites for teaching, the mere presence of the two does not guarantee an effective educator. Just as a world-class athlete may be a poor coach, a world-class surgeon may be an ineffective teacher. As such, surgeons must view teaching as another skill that needs to be developed and improved with time.

The Ethics of Surgical Training and Education

Particularly important to participating in surgical education is an understanding of the relevant ethics and ethical principles. The principle of non-maleficence (aka "do no harm") is a core component of the Hippocratic Oath. On an individual basis, a trainee performing a task (in or out of the operating room) theoretically places a patient at potential for greater harm when said task could be performed by someone more qualified [11]. From a societal perspective, we must each acknowledge and understand a desire for suitable care for others and for future generations of patients [11]. Patient-based medical and surgical education are a means of achieving this goal. Because of the limits of textbook learning or simulation training, teaching with patients will always be an integral part of surgeon education. Implicit with this social agreement, however, is the ethical responsibility of the medical educators to confirm that selection, instruction, and supervision of trainees protects the health and wellbeing of patients to a great degree [11].

It should be noted that participation of trainees does not necessarily lead to greater harm for patients. In a recent study examining data from the 2011 American College of Surgeons National Surgical Quality Improvement Program, orthopedic resident involvement during surgical procedures was associated with decreased morbidity and mortality [12]. While use of trainees may be associated with equivocal (or fewer) medical errors, time required to complete procedures is usually increased when working with a trainee. As such, there are opportunity costs from educating surgical trainees that could be done more efficiently by trained staff. With the increased emphasis on clinical productivity in the academic environment, surgical education tends to be one of the first casualties.

Being an Effective Surgical Educator

"Learn by doing" with an emphasis on volume has been a hallmark of traditional surgical training [13]. This traditional training adage is characteristic of a "pure discovery" model of learning. Pure discovery relies on the trainee to self-direct learning and concepts [14]. Although pure discovery systems require the least effort on the part of the educator, it is ultimately ineffective without appropriate explanation, focus, or feedback. Empirically this is true, because it is quite possible for a trainee to "go through the motions" of a procedure several times without ever fully grasping it conceptually or gaining the skill to perform it independently [15]. Observational studies of intraoperative learning note that when surgeons taught through instrumental actions without explanation or context, the learner is left to infer the lesson on their own [15].

More appropriate to modern surgical education is the guided discovery technique. The guided discovery model incorporates pre-task preparation, guidance during task completion, and debriefing after completion of the task. The guided discovery technique provides a more effective framework for learning and surgical skill acquisition when compared to a pure discovery technique [16]. Guided discovery is more time consuming for both the trainee and educator and requires commitment by both parties to succeed. Although we will focus on using the guided discovery model to facilitate intraoperative learning, it is applicable to any training environment. As such, the principles can be applied to teaching in the inpatient or ambulatory setting as well.

The first step in the guided discovered model involves the instructor framing the task at hand during preoperative discussion. This discussion may be formal or informal but is best when performed well in advance of a planned procedure. This discussion may include topics such as indications, learning goals, portions of the case that the trainee should be prepared to perform, and resources for further preparation. Preoperative counsel helps educators gain awareness and sensitivity to trainee learning needs, a trait associated with superior teachers [17]. Awareness of trainee knowledge and prior experience helps ensure that the teacher is able to challenge the trainee with new ideas, concepts, or tasks in a sense of graduated responsibility [18]. Trainees tend to have narrow learning goals for procedures when compared to those expressed by educators [19]. Preoperative conference can also help ensure that trainees maximize global learning as opposed to solely focusing on technical nuances.

While the guided discovery model requires more work on the part of the teacher, it also requires more effort on the learner as well. Setting clear expectations is important to ensure that each learning opportunity is not wasted. The learner is expected to come prepared to the operating room, to be aware of their limitations, and to be receptive to feedback. Preoperative counsel helps reinforce these expectations. With time, these expectations become ingrained in the culture of learning.

During the procedure, the teacher provides guidance to help the trainee complete the task(s). Maintaining composure is important to maximizing learning. Studies have demonstrated that trainees are more receptive to learning from teachers who are enthusiastic and remain calm and courteous, even in high stress situations [20]. Deconstruction of complex tasks into discernable motions or steps is particularly helpful to allow trainees to digest and process new items [18]. Complex tasks are more easily processed when they are presented with multiple sensory input. Surgeons are encouraged to verbalize their approach in addition to demonstrating it visually [21]. Haptic feedback is particularly helpful as well to learners processing new tasks. Trainees should be allowed to "feel the pathology" when possible. Including trainees in intraoperative decisions helps keep them engaged and can improve their surgical judgment [20].

Debriefing at the conclusion of the procedure solidifies the learning that occurred in the operation and helps guide future practice [14]. Debriefing entails providing thoughtful and considerate feedback. Feedback is a statement or gesture expressing positive (or negative) reaction to a behavior with the aim of increasing (or decreasing) the likelihood of that behavior happening again. Feedback is recognized as one of the most influential tools for learning in surgical training [22, 23]. When performed properly, feedback is efficient and promotes learner accountability, reflection, and self-assessment skills [24]. Perioperative feedback can have a direct translation to improved operative skills and has been associated with improvements in procedural errors, time, and economy of movement [25].

Despite this, feedback is frequently underutilized in the academic training environment [26]. When present, feedback is often limited, generic, pertinent to technical skills only, and infrequently suggests areas for improvement or formal action plans [24, 27].

Multiple standardized models have been created to facilitate regular, effective feedback [10, 14, 24]. Although each method varies in terms of its approach, there are many features of effective feedback that are independent of technique. Feedback should be undertaken with teacher and learner working as allies, with the common goal of improving learner performance and understanding. Effective feedback requires attention to incentives, timing, setting, and data. A safe learning environment is critical to promote an open, honest communication. It should be discussed temporally close to a behavior as possible so as to prevent recall bias. Feedback should also be expected on the part of the learner, so that they may be better prepared for self-reflection. Feedback should be specific, and supported by first-hand or objective data. It is most effective when it is regulated in quantity and focuses on remediable behaviors and actions.

We prefer to use the Ask-Tell-Ask (ATA) method for feedback. This standardized approach was originally developed at the Cleveland Clinic to enhance physician-patient communication [24, 28]. The ATA method is a learner-centered approach comprised of three steps for reinforcing and modifying behaviors. In step one, the teacher asks the learner for a self-assessment of their performance using non-judgmental, open-ended questions such as "What went well and what could have gone better?" In step two, the teacher should address the student's assessment and acknowledge any concerns the learner expressed. The teacher should state at least one thing that the learner did well and discuss potential areas or improvement based on their observations. Teachers should use the term "and" instead of "but" when performing this step. "And" lowers cognitive resistance, whereas "but" tends to mitigate achievement and prompts the student to plan a rebuttal. This discussion should be interactive, allowing the student to reflect on things that could have been done differently. It is important to limit areas of improvement to one to two items to prevent the student from becoming overwhelmed. In step three, the teacher confirms the student's understanding and works with them to formulate an action plan for improvement moving forward [24]. The ATA is quick, reliable, and applicable in multiple settings.

Simulation and the Future of Orthopedic Education

Surgical simulation is relatively new paradigm in surgical education [29]. Numerous platforms exist including synthetic bone models, cadaver laboratory sessions, computer software programs, and computerized simulator machines [29]. Simulation provides a safe, stress-free platform for learning without the potential for patient harm. Simulation also presents the opportunity for uniform educational experience that is absent in patient-based experiences. As such, simulation also allows for more standardized assessment of trainee performance [30].

Interest in simulation-based surgical training methods has increased significantly over the past decade. Orthopedic residency program directors and residents have agreed that surgical skills laboratories and simulator technology should be a required component of orthopedic resident training [31]. Numerous high fidelity and low fidelity simulation systems for surgical training have been developed. The high fidelity systems promote more advanced features and realism often at a significantly higher cost. Low fidelity systems tend to be less refined, more portable, and aimed at teaching basic surgical skills. Interestingly, high fidelity and low fidelity simulation systems seem to have similar results.

There is a small, but enlarging body of evidence that suggests that simulation technology can improve trainee skill. The majority of this evidence is in general surgery literature, particularly with respect to laparoscopic skills. The implication of these studies is that simulation may decrease intraoperative time, cost, errors, and patient morbidity. In the orthopedic literature, simulation modules have demonstrated short-term improvement in a wide variety of tasks including microvascular skills [32], short arm casting [33], Pavlik harness application [34], and arthroscopic Bankart repair [35].

Although simulation offers great potential to enhance trainee learning, there are many limitations to this technology. A lack of funding has been cited as the biggest barrier to the widespread adoption of surgical skills laboratories and simulator trainers [31]. In light of these financial challenges, lower fidelity methods have become quite popular and seem to serve a similar purpose to high fidelity simulators in modern-day orthopedic education. Trainees note that many simulators, high fidelity models, lack realism. This lack of perceived realism is particularly true with respect to haptic feedback [29]. The real world transfer of technical skills learnt from simulators is less consistent for open surgical procedures when compared to endoscopic or arthroscopic modes [36]. Furthermore, although simulators provide the opportunity to teach discrete technical skills, teaching surgical judgment and intraoperative decision making still requires significant teacher feedback and involvement [27, 37]. While simulation may build repeatable skills, it does not mirror the stresses of the operative environment; it is simply another avenue to build technique performance.

In the current residency training model, trainees have a limited amount of time to utilize simulation training resources due to patient care responsibilities. Last but not least, simulation resources may be very expensive and in some cases are not renewable. For these reasons and more, simulation should be viewed as an augment to actual operative exposure, not as a potential replacement.

Conclusion

Surgical education has evolved significantly over the past centuries. Despite challenges to education, there are numerous ethical, personal, and professional incentives for surgeons to engage in teaching. The guided discovery model incorporates pre-task preparation, guidance during task completion, and debriefing after completion of the task. The guided discovery model is the most effective way to teach surgical skills and is simple, quick, and easy to incorporate in daily surgical practice. Surgical simulation has been shown to improve trainee skill outside of the operating room and has potential to complement trainee education in the future.

References

1. Wilson FC. Residents as teachers. J Bone Joint Surg Am. 2001;83-A(9):1441–3.
2. Emery SE, Guss D, Kuremsky MA, Hamlin BR, Herndon JH, Rubash HE. Resident education versus fellowship training-conflict or synergy? AOA critical issues. J Bone Joint Surg Am. 2012;94(21):e159.
3. Langsley DG. Medical specialty credentialing in the United States. Clin Orthop Relat Res. 1990;(257):22–8.
4. History of the American Board of Orthopedic Surgery 2017 [cited 2017 January 10]. Available from: https://www.abos.org/about-abos/history.aspx.
5. Peabody TD. Those who can, do-those who can, teach: AOA critical issues. J Bone Joint Surg Am. 2013;95(19):e1431–3.
6. Levine WN, Spang RC. ACGME duty hour requirements: perceptions and impact on resident training and patient care. J Am Acad Orthop Surg. 2014;22(9):535–44.
7. Baskies MA, Ruchelsman DE, Capeci CM, Zuckerman JD, Egol KA. Operative experience in an Orthopedic surgery residency program: the effect of work-hour restrictions. J Bone Joint Surg Am. 2008;90(4):924–7.
8. Pappas AJ, Teague DC. The impact of the accreditation council for graduate medical education work-hour regulations on the surgical experience of Orthopedic surgery residents. J Bone Joint Surg Am. 2007;89(4):904–9.
9. Choma NN, Vasilevskis EE, Sponsler KC, Hathaway J, Kripalani S. Effect of the ACGME 16-hour rule on efficiency and quality of care: duty hours 2.0. JAMA Intern Med. 2013;173(9):819–21.
10. Ahmed M, Arora S, Russ S, Darzi A, Vincent C, Sevdalis N. Operation debrief: a SHARP improvement in performance feedback in the operating room. Ann Surg. 2013;258(6):958–63.
11. Capozzi JD, Rhodes R. Residency training. J Bone Joint Surg Am. 2000;82(9):1356–7.
12. Edelstein AI, Lovecchio FC, Saha S, Hsu WK, Kim JY. Impact of resident involvement on Orthopedic surgery outcomes: an analysis of 30,628 patients from the American College of Surgeons National Surgical Quality Improvement Program Database. J Bone Joint Surg Am. 2014;96(15):e131.
13. Reznick RK, MacRae H. Teaching surgical skills--changes in the wind. N Engl J Med. 2006;355(25):2664–9.
14. Roberts NK, Williams RG, Kim MJ, Dunnington GL. The briefing, intraoperative teaching, debriefing model for teaching in the operating room. J Am Coll Surg. 2009;208(2):299–303.
15. Roberts NK, Brenner MJ, Williams RG, Kim MJ, Dunnington GL. Capturing the teachable moment: a grounded theory study of verbal teaching interactions in the operating room. Surgery. 2012;151(5):643–50.

16. Mayer RE. Should there be a three-strikes rule against pure discovery learning? the case for guided methods of instruction. Am Psychol. 2004;59(1):14–9.
17. Cox SS, Swanson MS. Identification of teaching excellence in operating room and clinic settings. Am J Surg. 2002;183(3):251–5.
18. Blom EM, Verdaasdonk EG, Stassen LP, Stassen HG, Wieringa PA, Dankelman J. Analysis of verbal communication during teaching in the operating room and the potentials for surgical training. Surg Endosc. 2007;21(9):1560–6.
19. Pernar LI, Breen E, Ashley SW, Peyre SE. Preoperative learning goals set by surgical residents and faculty. J Surg Res. 2011;170(1):1–5.
20. Iwaszkiewicz M, Darosa DA, Risucci DA. Efforts to enhance operating room teaching. J Surg Educ. 2008;65(6):436–40.
21. Snyder RA, Tarpley MJ, Tarpley JL, Davidson M, Brophy C, Dattilo JB. Teaching in the operating room: results of a national survey. J Surg Educ. 2012;69(5):643–9.
22. Jensen AR, Wright AS, Kim S, Horvath KD, Calhoun KE. Educational feedback in the operating room: a gap between resident and faculty perceptions. Am J Surg. 2012;204(2):248–55.
23. El Boghdady M, Alijani A. Feedback in surgical education. Surgeon. 2017;15(2):98–103.
24. French JC, Colbert CY, Pien LC, Dannefer EF, Taylor CA. Targeted feedback in the milestones era: utilization of the ask-tell-ask feedback model to promote reflection and self-assessment. J Surg Educ. 2015;72(6):e274–9.
25. Grantcharov TP, Schulze S, Kristiansen VB. The impact of objective assessment and constructive feedback on improvement of laparoscopic performance in the operating room. Surg Endosc. 2007;21(12):2240–3.
26. Ahmed M, Sevdalis N, Vincent C, Arora S. Actual vs perceived performance debriefing in surgery: practice far from perfect. Am J Surg. 2013;205(4):434–40.
27. McKendy KM, Watanabe Y, Lee L, Bilgic E, Enani G, Feldman LS, et al. Perioperative feedback in surgical training: a systematic review. Am J Surg. 2017;214(1):117–26.
28. Barnett PB. Rapport and the hospitalist. Am J Med. 2001;111(9B):31S–5S.
29. Atesok K, Mabrey JD, Jazrawi LM, Egol KA. Surgical simulation in Orthopedic skills training. J Am Acad Orthop Surg. 2012;20(7):410–22.
30. Michelson JD. Simulation in Orthopedic education: an overview of theory and practice. J Bone Joint Surg Am. 2006;88(6):1405–11.
31. Karam MD, Pedowitz RA, Natividad H, Murray J, Marsh JL. Current and future use of surgical skills training laboratories in Orthopedic resident education: a national survey. J Bone Joint Surg Am. 2013;95(1):e4.
32. Ko JW, Lorzano A, Mirarchi AJ. Effectiveness of a microvascular surgery training curriculum for Orthopedic surgery residents. J Bone Joint Surg Am. 2015;97(11):950–5.
33. Moktar J, Popkin CA, Howard A, Murnaghan ML. Development of a cast application simulator and evaluation of objective measures of performance. J Bone Joint Surg Am. 2014;96(9):e76.
34. Moktar J, Bradley CS, Maxwell A, Wedge JH, Kelley SP, Murnaghan ML. Skill acquisition and retention following simulation-based training in Pavlik harness application. J Bone Joint Surg Am. 2016;98(10):866–70.
35. Howells NR, Auplish S, Hand GC, Gill HS, Carr AJ, Rees JL. Retention of arthroscopic shoulder skills learned with use of a simulator. Demonstration of a learning curve and loss of performance level after a time delay. J Bone Joint Surg Am. 2009;91(5):1207–13.
36. Fonseca AL, Evans LV, Gusberg RJ. Open surgical simulation in residency training: a review of its status and a case for its incorporation. J Surg Educ. 2013;70(1):129–37.
37. Andersen DK. How can educators use simulation applications to teach and assess surgical judgment? Acad Med. 2012;87(7):934–41.

Chapter 13
Independent Medical Examinations and Legal Depositions

Fady Y. Hijji, Ankur S. Narain, Krishna T. Kudaravalli, Kelly H. Yom, Edward Goldberg, and Kern Singh

Introduction

Approximately 40% of chronic conditions, 54% of long-term disabilities, and 24% of activity restricted days are attributable to musculoskeletal conditions and injuries [1]. Furthermore, musculoskeletal pathologies are responsible for more than half of all absences lasting 2 weeks or longer, making it a primary cause for workplace absence in industrialized countries [2, 3]. As a result of this productivity loss, these disabilities also lead to significant indirect costs. Workers' compensation was originally developed to assist those who are injured or fall ill as a result of their occupation and also to serve as a method of cost control [4, 5]. However, in order to adequately establish a patient's level of disability and to identify a patient's ability to return to gainful employment, independent medical examinations (IMEs) were established.

IMEs are performed by medical practitioners including, but not limited to, physicians, dentists, or chiropractors who are not otherwise involved in the typical direct care or treatment of the patient [5]. Oftentimes, these healthcare professionals perform the examinations at the request of the patient's employer and less frequently for the worker's representation. During the IME, a formal assessment is made determining the general health of the patient, documenting all injuries and illnesses, and elucidating potential associations between the injury or illness and the patient's work or work environment [6].

Through the utilization of an IME, the medical practitioner is able to provide an objective analysis of a patient's health [5]. Additionally, contracting physicians through a third party is thought to limit the patient-physician relationship [7]. Despite these safeguards, the engagement of an IME physician through a worker's compensation insurance carrier or employer may lead to a formation of inherent

F. Y. Hijji · A. S. Narain · K. T. Kudaravalli · K. H. Yom · E. Goldberg · K. Singh (✉)
Department of Orthopedic Surgery, Rush University Medical Center, Chicago, IL, USA
e-mail: kkudar2@illinois.edu; egoldberg@rushortho.com; kern.singh@rushortho.com

E. C. Makhni et al. (eds.), *Orthopedic Practice Management*,
https://doi.org/10.1007/978-3-319-96938-1_13

biases [4, 8]. The purpose of this chapter is to discuss the history, guidelines, principles, potential conflicts, and limitations regarding IMEs and legal depositions.

History of Independent Medical Examinations

The Progressive Era of the early 1900s represented a period during which significant interest was placed on workplace injuries and deaths [5]. During this time, there was also increasing attention toward the welfare of the working lower class, minorities, and women. As a result, states began enacting the first laws to protect the rights of workers and implement work safety and compensation for injury. In 1902, Maryland became the first state to pass a worker's compensation law [9]. In 1908, the first federal regulation regarding worker's compensation was instituted, along with multiple protective labor laws including the Federal Employers Liability Act [9]. This labor law protected railroad workers from potential negligence on the part of employers, and similar laws for different occupations shortly followed.

Following the establishment of many labor and federal worker's compensation laws, worker's compensation groups began to form. The American College of Occupational and Environmental Medicine (ACOEM) was founded by surgeons with the goal to reduce the risk of work-related injury and illness in the population [5]. Members of this group identified a variety of work-related factors that were associated with an increased risk for injury and provided public education regarding these hazards [5]. This group would also go on to establish some of the guidelines utilized for modern IMEs.

Although many work-related hazards and injuries were reported with increasing frequency, workers were still incapable of receiving the funds necessary for their medical treatment and subsequent compensation. In 1970, the Occupational Safety and Health Act was established to further support the injured worker [9]. It was at this time that workers obtained many of the rights necessary to litigate their claims in court. This act would eventually lead the way toward the development of IMEs.

Utility of IME and Depositions

In the setting of an injured worker, an appropriate assessment is required to determine if a correlation exists between the injury and the work environment. Additionally, it is necessary to assess the degree of disability associated with the injury and to determine the estimated time required before the individual can return to work. IMEs provide the medical context of the injury, the appropriateness of past and future treatment, as well as determine the extent of injury. Through this independent and objective assessment, both workers and employers can potentially benefit [2, 4, 5].

IMEs potentially protect the worker by identifying the level of disability and directing necessary compensation and treatment [10]. Following an injury, IMEs can identify the pathology responsible for the injury and the association of the injury to the work environment [6]. By providing evidence of work-related injury, the worker is capable of seeking the appropriate compensation and treatment. A physician's medical opinion is also required for an insurance provider to deny a claim, which prevents employers or insurers from inappropriately denying potential compensation for a worker's injury [11]. Finally, the thorough history and physical examinations performed during IMEs allow for the identification of predictive factors for long-term disability, such as fear avoidance and depression [5]. As such, a patient can be directed toward the treatment necessary to maximize the likelihood of successful long-term outcomes.

Guidelines of IME and the Controversy

A physician adheres to a variety of guidelines when performing an IME [5]. These guidelines are predominantly established by various federal regulations as defined by the Social Security Administration, as well as local state laws [5]. Medical organizations also contribute to many IME guidelines, such as the American Medical Association's (AMA) Guidelines to the Evaluation of Permanent Impairment [5]. These guidelines have been established as the legal standard in determining the degree of disability. The American College of Surgeons has also established supplementary guidelines to aid the physician in performing an IME [12, 13]. In general, these guidelines provide methods for measuring functional impairment and disability. They also guide physicians in assessing mental and social impairment and performing musculoskeletal examinations.

Despite the official sources of established IME guidelines, concern exists regarding the objectivity of these guidelines. Frequently, occupational medicine guidelines are sponsored by pharmaceutical and medical device manufacturers [5]. This sponsorship inevitably raises concerns regarding the influence of corporate interests on IME guidelines [14]. ACOEM has previously been noted to exhibit many of these potential conflicts of interest [14]. Multiple members who serve on the guidelines committee have reported relationships with industry, potentially using their place on the committee for financial gain [14]. Furthermore, many committee members have demonstrated minimal expertise on the relevant subjects for these guidelines [5]. Although these guidelines exhibit some potential for conflicts of interest, the guidelines for IMEs and medicolegal opinions are often compared to those utilized for clinical practice [5]. This prevents bias from impacting specific guidelines or causing deviation from medical standards.

Qualifications of Medical Experts

The physician performing an IME is known as a medical expert witness. However, it is important to note that in the legal setting, an expert may simply be a specialized physician, rather than an expert as defined by their peers [7]. As such, a variety of medical societies have established a range of qualifications that a physician must exhibit in order to conduct IMEs. Primarily, the physician performing an IME must be in current practice with active involvement with patients similar to those receiving the IME [15]. If the physician is not in active practice, they must be capable of demonstrating competence within the relevant field. In order to demonstrate this competence, the expert witness must be capable of citing relevant publications, or must demonstrate recent involvement with teaching of medical trainees [7]. Additionally, the American College of Surgeons has stated that the expert witness must be prepared to explain the basis of their opinion following provision of their testimony [16]. This can include personal experience, specific literature, established evidence-based guidelines, or other experts' opinions.

It is also recommended that the medical expert have a familiarity with the AMA Guidelines to the Evaluation of Permanent Impairment, as this is the legal standard in many individual states [6]. Additionally, a physician may choose to complete a course and subsequent examination administered by the American Board of Independent Medical Examiners, allowing them to obtain a certification to perform IMEs [5].

The Process for Conducting an IME

Preliminary Phase

When offered an assignment for an IME, it is crucial for the physician to review all aspects of the case [6]. The appropriateness and time frame of the case, as well as the questions being asked, are all factors to be considered [6]. Prior to the examination, the physician should take the time to orient the patient regarding the purpose of the examination. The patient should also be encouraged to provide the most honest and accurate representation of their history and symptoms. Additionally, it is crucial to inform the patient that the physician-patient relationship with IMEs differs from the standard, wherein the examination is not confidential and there is limited disclosure of medical observations to the patient [6].

Patient Interview and History

A substantial amount of important information can be obtained from the patient history during an IME. How the patient relays the history is as important as the information contained within the history [6]. In the situation of an injury or impairment, understanding how a patient has responded to the injury can be helpful in determining a patient's impairment [6]. Additionally, it is important to elucidate patient social and occupational responsibilities [17]. As such, it is crucial for the physician to utilize critical observation during history-taking. This requires taking note of the emotional and cognitive state, language skills, and the demeanor of the patient at the time of the interview as well as the conditions in which the interview was conducted [6].

In addition to the standard medical history, it is important for the physician to inquire about a variety of personal and familial factors that may serve as sources for patient distress [5]. Marital status, number of dependents within the household, and familial health are all potential topics that may be covered during the interview. Furthermore, inquiring about social history may identify potential drug abuse or physical abuse that can contribute to a patient's symptoms [18]. These factors have previously been noted to occur in over 60% of patients with chronic pain [18].

Finally, a physician should obtain an understanding of the event resulting in the relevant injury. However, in order to best utilize this information, physicians participating in IMEs should be comfortable with the biomechanics involved in common orthopedic injuries [6]. By understanding these basic mechanisms, a physician can gain an appreciation for the relevance of certain events on the chief complaint or disability [6].

Physical Examination

Following the patient history, a physical examination is performed. For orthopedic surgeons, it is often necessary to perform a thorough musculoskeletal and neurologic examination in order to identify the true degree of injury and impairment [19]. In addition to the physical examination, many examiners frequently utilize validated surveys to measure baseline functional status and disability [6]. During the examination phase of the IME, it is crucial that the physician take note of any inconsistencies with patient responses and lack of effort during physical examination maneuvers.

Review of Documentation

In order to provide a thorough evaluation, the examiner must review all available medical records and documentation. The combination of the clinical evaluation with the information provided by relevant documentation, such as previous notes from other caregivers or examiners, can highlight discordance within a patient's functional status [6]. While subjective differences may occur between clinicians, it is not expected for there to be substantial differences among physical examination findings or the patient's reported history.

The timing for reviewing this information is at the discretion of the evaluator. Analyzing previous records and laboratory tests prior to the IME may identify questions that should be addressed during the interview [6].

Following the evaluation, the physician may choose to request additional information if necessary. Occasionally, the provided documentation is not sufficient to produce a thorough evaluation [6]. In this situation, the physician can request further imaging studies or interventions. For example, a patient presenting with chronic fatigue following an accident may in fact be suffering from sleep apnea. As such, a sleep study may be necessary if one has not been done prior to the IME assignment.

Preparing the Report

Upon completion of the examination, the report discussing the clinician's impressions, diagnoses, and recommendations is compiled. When presenting relevant impressions and conclusions, the physician should identify the relative strength of each medical opinion [6]. By stratifying conclusions as probable (greater than 50% chance that the injury is related to a work incident) or possible (less than 50% chance), a medical examiner can characterize a claim's credibility [5]. The physician can then provide professional opinions regarding necessary medical care in the future, as well as work restrictions as related to the claim. Additionally, a physician can stratify medical impressions into injury-related and non-injury-related categories [6]. This can facilitate the reader's understanding and ensure that all relevant questions are answered. For the sake of completeness, examiners will also typically provide opinions on maximum medical improvement (MMI) for the relevant injuries or disabilities [6]. Injury prognosis and the ability to return to work will also be mentioned in the reports.

Testimony

The examiner will often be required to present their findings during a deposition or testimony in court. During this legal process, it is crucial for the physician to remain impartial [7]. The examiner should be objective in the medical assessment of a case, especially in the presence of differing opinions from colleagues. Additionally, prior to the deposition, physicians should ensure up-to-date knowledge on relevant literature and review all notes and reports to avoid conflicting statements [6].

Doctor-Patient Relationship in IMEs

The doctor-patient relationship in an IME differs from that in a standard clinical setting [10]. Typically, a physician forms an implied contract when agreeing to enter a professional relationship with a patient who is seeking treatment [20]. Due to the fact that there is no intention to treat the patient, the physician exhibits a different role with different responsibilities. For example, the physician performing an IME may not be obligated to disclose findings or impressions with the patient. In fact, the referring party oftentimes maintains the release of this information [21, 22].

Due to the limited relationship between an examiner and a patient during an IME, the examiner's liability remains questionable [7, 10]. Some courts have argued that a physician does not have the full obligation to disclose treatment to the patient during an IME [21]. However, previous courts have also declared that, in specific situations, the limited relationship still requires the physician to uphold certain standards. A physician may be held accountable if a patient is injured during the examination, or if they fail to disclose critical medical information that indicate a serious or life-threatening condition [10]. For example, in a case in 2004, the Arizona Supreme Court determined that a radiologist may be liable for failing to inform a patient of findings indicative of a life-threatening condition, despite having only been requested to review a chest X-ray for an IME-relevant tuberculosis screening [10]. As such, a physician performing an IME should disclose significant life-threatening medical findings to a patient and suggest that they seek medical care regardless of its relation to the IME.

Conflicts of Interest in Medicolegal Practice

A conflict of interest (COI) occurs when a physician's judgment or actions are influenced by a secondary gain [7]. However, in order for a COI to exist, a secondary interest with the potential to affect a physician's actions must be present [23]. In the context of IMEs, a COI may affect the physician's ability to remain objective when providing a professional opinion or giving testimony [7]. As such, it is important to be aware of the potential sources for COIs when performing an IME.

Depending on a physician's intentions for performing an IME, a variety of COIs can exist. Previous sources have noted that non-monetary benefits can be obtained from performing IMEs, such as increasing a physician's reputation [24]. Additionally, participating in IMEs offers an opportunity to serve the public, and provides an incentive to stay up to date with the relevant literature [7].

A physician performing an IME is typically compensated for the examination, record reviews, and depositions. Due to the fact that IMEs are typically requested by the respondent, there is pressure on the physician to provide medical impressions in favor of the employer or insurer [7]. Environments such as these have led some critics to state that IME physicians have often decided their position prior to analyzing the findings and evidence [7]. However, by following the appropriate guidelines and staying within the limits of professional knowledge and experience, a physician has the ability to remain impartial [7].

The Adversarial System

Despite the potential biases that exist during IMEs, the adversary theory claims that these biases should even out [7]. COIs may exist on both sides of any case, but through cross examination or the utilization of two opposing experts, the potential biases are thought to balance each other. In this situation, objective evidence would prevail in determining the final outcome of any given case.

In an ideal setting, a single objective examiner would be sufficient to present the medical evidence necessary for a court to render a decision. As such, two opposing experts can be utilized to present their own evidence, and these opinions can be weighed against the potential biases. In addition to potential conflicts, an examiner's presentation and opinion will be largely dependent on the questions posed by the attorneys during trials and depositions. Due to the adversarial system, a case's outcome is largely dictated by the attorneys' abilities rather than the expertise of the examiner [7]. As such, it is the responsibility of the attorneys for both parties to utilize questions that support their respective positions. The expert witness will be required to answer truthfully for both parties, using only evidence-based medicine and clinical expertise to support their answers. This can further assist in mitigating the effects of bias on medical impressions or testimonies [7].

Continuing Education for Medical Experts

Many of the limitations within IMEs can be stymied by the utilization of evidence-based medicine. A substantial amount of information that physicians learn during training becomes outdated over time, as much of this knowledge is typically based on anecdotal evidence or experience [7]. In order to adequately care for patients, physicians must keep current with the literature. Similarly, in order to appropriately perform an IME, a physician must be able to demonstrate familiarity with up-to-date practices and new concepts [5]. A medical opinion and subsequent testimony provided by an examiner should be consistent with standards of care, capable of undergoing the scrutiny of other experts within the field [6].

However, the effect of learning theory may inhibit some physicians from changing their practices to newer standards. Some physicians hold on to outdated theories and practices due to the belief that "things learned first are things learned best" [7]. Consequently, physicians participating in IMEs may provide expert opinions despite not having been formally introduced to recent guidelines and updated practices. Due to the lack of feedback associated with IMEs, a physician may continue providing this type of information without self-correction [7]. In order to prevent this, many medical societies now subject expert opinions to peer review and are able to file complaints against potentially biased or unethical testimony [7]. As such, physicians performing IMEs should continue to follow the necessary guidelines and remain familiar with the recent literature and standards of care.

Summary

Work-related injuries and illness are a common source of disability and productivity loss among the working class. IMEs have been developed with the goal of protecting workers subjected to harm in the workplace, while also serving as a method to provide fair and just treatment to injured workers. In order to adequately perform an IME and objectively analyze a worker's claim, a physician must adhere to a variety of medical guidelines and be able to provide evidence-based medical opinions. The limited relationship that exists between a physician and a patient during an IME facilitates the objective medical evaluation of a patient. However, this limited relationship has also served as a source of controversy due to potential conflicts of interest and questionable physician liability. A physician performing an IME must be able to provide a thorough and objective medical evaluation and remain familiar with current medical literature in order to avoid conflicts with the patient, employer, and healthcare system.

Disclosure No funds were received in support of this work. No benefits in any form have been or will be received from any commercial party related directly or indirectly to the subject of this manuscript.

References

1. Badley EM, Rasooly I, Webster GK. Relative importance of musculoskeletal disorders as a cause of chronic health problems, disability, and health care utilization: findings from the 1990 Ontario health survey. J Rheumatol. 1994;21(3):505–14.
2. Clifton DW Jr. The functional IME: a linkage of expertise across the disability continuum. Work. 2006;26(3):281–5.
3. Brage S, Nygard JF, Tellnes G. The gender gap in musculoskeletal-related long-term sickness absence in Norway. Scand J Soc Med. 1998;26(1):34–43.
4. Lax M. Independent of what? The independent medical examination business. New Solut. 2004;14(3):219–51.
5. Ky P, Hameed H, Christo PJ. Independent medical examinations: facts and fallacies. Pain Physician. 2009;12(5):811–8.
6. Ameis A, Zasler ND. The independent medical examination. Phys Med Rehabil Clin N Am. 2002;13(2):259–86. ix
7. Schofferman J. Opinions and testimony of expert witnesses and independent medical evaluators. Pain Med. 2007;8(4):376–82.
8. Morton WE. In response to the 2002, vol. 22, no. 4 article entitled the rise and fall of occupational medicine in the United States. Am J Prev Med. 2002;23(4):309.
9. Aldrich M. Safety first: technology, labor, and business in the building of work safety. Baltimore, Maryland: Johns Hopkins University Press; 1997.
10. Baum K. Independent medical examinations: an expanding source of physician liability. Ann Intern Med. 2005;142(12 Pt 1):974–8.
11. Heilbronner RL. Independent medical evaluation. In: Kreutzer JS, DeLuca J, Caplan B, editors. Encyclopedia of clinical neuropsychology. New York: Springer New York; 2011. p. 1305–6.
12. Trescot AM, Boswell MV, Atluri SL, et al. Opioid guidelines in the management of chronic non-cancer pain. Pain Physician. 2006;9(1):1–39.

13. Manchikanti L, Abdi S, Atluri S, et al. An update of comprehensive evidence-based guidelines for interventional techniques in chronic spinal pain. Part II: guidance and recommendations. Pain Physician. 2013;16(2 Suppl):S49–283.
14. Manchikanti L, Singh V, Derby R, et al. Review of occupational medicine practice guidelines for interventional pain management and potential implications. Pain Physician. 2008;11(3):271–89.
15. Williams MA, Mackin GA, Beresford HR, et al. American academy of neurology qualifications and guidelines for the physician expert witness. Neurology. 2006;66(1):13–4.
16. Patient S, Professional Liability Committee of the American College of S. Statement on the physician acting as an expert witness. Bull Am Coll Surg. 2011;96(4):39–40.
17. van der Giezen AM, Bouter LM, Nijhuis FJ. Prediction of return-to-work of low back pain patients sicklisted for 3-4 months. Pain. 2000;87(3):285–94.
18. Bailey BE, Freedenfeld RN, Kiser RS, Gatchel RJ. Lifetime physical and sexual abuse in chronic pain patients: psychosocial correlates and treatment outcomes. Disabil Rehabil. 2003;25(7):331–42.
19. Koppenhoefer RM. In: Delisa JA, editor. Disability evaluation in rehabilitation medicine: principles and practice. Philadelphia: Lippincott; 1988.
20. Suk M, Udale AM, Helfet DL. Orthopaedics and the law. J Am Acad Orthop Surg. 2005;13(6):397–406.
21. Ebrahim S, Sava H, Kunz R, Busse JW. Ethics and legalities associated with independent medical evaluations. CMAJ. 2014;186(4):248–9.
22. Grant D. Independent medical examinations and the fuzzy politics of disclosure. CMAJ. 1997;156(1):73–5.
23. Camilleri M, Gamble GL, Kopecky SL, Wood MB, Hockema ML. Principles and process in the development of the Mayo Clinic's individual and institutional conflict of interest policy. Mayo Clin Proc. 2005;80(10):1340–6.
24. Ashar BH, Miller RG, Powe NR. Extent and determinants of physician participation in expert witness testimony. South Med J. 2005;98(4):444–9.

Chapter 14
Board Certification and Maintenance in Orthopedic Surgery

Kenneth R. Gundle

An Overview of the American Board of Orthopedic Surgery

Purpose

The mission of the ABOS is to ensure the safe, ethical, and effective practice of orthopedic surgery for the public benefit, through standards for education, practice, and conduct [1]. It does so through its involvement in residency education requirements, and in particular through its programs for certification and maintenance of certification. While it is individual state medical boards that grant a license to practice medicine, the ABOS allows those who practice orthopedic surgery to obtain an additional designation as being board certified. While technically optional, many hospitals and other organizations prefer or require orthopedic surgeons to be either eligible for boards certification, or already certified. In this manner, the ABOS serves as a self-governance organization for the practice of orthopedic surgery in the United States.

History

The ABOS was formed in the 1930s as both American medicine and orthopedics were making a fundamental transformation [2]. The American Orthopedic Association (AOA) had been established in 1887 and was the first formally

K. R. Gundle
Orthopedic Oncology, Orgeon Health and Science University, Department of Orthopedics and Rehabilitation, Portland VA Medical Center, Operative Care Division, Portland, OR, USA
e-mail: gundle@oshu.edu

E. C. Makhni et al. (eds.), *Orthopedic Practice Management*,
https://doi.org/10.1007/978-3-319-96938-1_14

organized body representing orthopedic surgery. The AOA served in part to provide a measure of one's acceptance as an orthopedic surgeon, as membership required several years of practice focusing on orthopedics as well as presenting at its annual meeting. In part to provide an organization with a broader member base, the American Academy of Orthopedic Surgeons (AAOS) was formed in 1933. That same year, the AOA recommended the formation of a specialty board to certify orthopedic surgeons, made up of representatives of the AOA, the AAOS, and the orthopedic surgeon section of the American Medical Association [3]. By the following year the ABOS was incorporated, and in 1936 it published formal requirements for certification. The ABOS is a member of the American Board of Medical Specialties.

The certification requirements at the time the ABOS was founded involved no particular examination or ongoing maintenance. However, applicants were required to have graduated from an AMA approved medical school, have a license to practice in the state of residency, and be an AMA or other approved society member in addition to upholding high ethical and professional standards. Subsequent requirements for a period of residency and independent practice were soon added.

Structure of the ABOS

The ABOS is a nonprofit, autonomous, private organization. Candidates who volunteer for evaluation are reviewed by the Board, and the Board sets the standards for issuing certifications [4]. It also works alongside the Accreditation Council for Graduate Medical Education's (ACGME) Residency Review Committee (RRC) in defining minimal educational standards for orthopedic training [3].

The current structure of the ABOS connects directly to its origin. The Directors are all diplomates, and are elected by ballot slates proposed by three organizations: the AOA, the AAOS, and the AMA Council of Medical Education. The ABOS Directors serve without compensation [4].

How the ABOS Is Different from the AOA and the AAOS

The mission of the ABOS is distinct than the AOA or AAOS. Its purpose is to ensure safe and effective practice of orthopedic surgery for the public benefit, through participating in setting regulations for training and through its certification programs. The AOA is a limited membership organization that is focused on engaging the orthopedic community in developing the leaders, strategies, and resources to help guide the future of musculoskeletal care. Membership is itself an accomplishment, with elected members expected to be accomplished in several domains of leadership, scholarship, and engagement. The AAOS is also a membership organization, with a focus on providing extensive education and practice management services broadly to the field of orthopedics. Application to become a fellow of the AAOS is open to all trained board-certified orthopedic surgeons. Through its Association and political action committee, the AAOS is also significantly involved in representing orthopedic surgeons in the health policy and regulation advocacy arena. If one were to make a *loose* comparison to the federal United States political structure, the AAOS would represent the House of Representatives (and somewhat the Executive branch), the AOA is rather akin to the Senate, and the ABOS is something between the Judiciary (although each organization has membership review mechanisms) and a regulatory agency.

Board Certification

Overview

While time-consuming and stressful for those going through the certification process or trying to squeeze in Maintenance of Certification (MOC) requirements, board certification in orthopedic surgery has a very rational structure. The formal process begins with a cognitive examination of medical knowledge at the completion of residency training (Part I), and is then followed by a review of candidates' own cases through formal oral case presentations and examination by established diplomates (Part II). Ongoing learning and practice quality is assessed through an organized MOC program.

Part I

The Part I examination is not a focus of this chapter, as residents take this at the conclusion of residency before starting fellowship or independent practice. Its structure is also more familiar to US-trained physicians, due to myriad other multiple choice–based examinations throughout schooling and training. The examination's structure and related literature will be briefly reviewed.

Structure

Part I is a cognitive examination spanning the breath of orthopedic surgery. It is designed to have approximately one-third of questions relate to basic science topics [5]. Care is taken to keep the test of similar difficulty year to year, and about one-third of the questions reportedly come from previous examinations. This examination is not graded "on the curve." Rather it is criterion-referenced, and it is indeed possible for everyone taking it to pass [6]. From 2012 to 2016, the overall failure rate ranged from 10% to 15%, though for first-time test takers it was between 4% and 7% [7].

The process of creating the examination is formal and time-consuming. The written examination is created by over 40 orthopedic surgeons from around the United States, and the work begins 2 years prior to the examination [5]. By the time a question is used at examination it has gone through five levels of editing, and questions are re-edited every 3–5 years on a rolling basis [6]. One practical result of this laborious process is that it is unlikely that any new literature from within the past year, and certainly not in the past 6 months, would be specifically tested.

After the examination, scores are evaluated for their psychometric properties, and questions considered defective based on psychometrics are removed. It is this process that prevents immediate release of the scores. So as another practical point, if there is a question you just think is wrong, or the right answer not present, it may be better to just move knowing it could ultimately be removed from the examination and unscored.

What We Know About Predictors of Success and Failure in Part I

The question of predictors for passing Part I has been examined by multiple authors. For example, a single large residency program with 19 Part I failures over 15 years noted that residents who failed Part I had lower OITE scores, lower USMLE Step I scores, less honors designation during medical school clinical rotations, and a weaker Deans letter [8]. Another study which examined four programs also noted a moderate correlation between Part 1 scores and both USMLE Step 1 scores and OITE scores (more so in later years of residency) [9]. The practical lesson for residents is that studying for the OITE each year indeed seems to be good preparation for Part I.

Part II

> What could be more valid than examining a candidate with use of his or her own cases? It is truly the best way to measure practice performance. [5]

Part II is designed as a practice-based oral examination. It is meant to assess one's ability to apply in clinical practice the cognitive knowledge tested in Part I. Candidates report all cases to the ABOS for a 6-month period (currently April through September) with diagnoses, procedure codes, and a brief description via an online portal called Scribe. The case lists are finalized by October 31; they are then reviewed by the ABOS and 12 cases are selected for formal presentation. These oral presentations are structured like case conferences during residency, with a summary provided by the candidate, who then responds to questions posed by examiners. Candidates may select a specific subspecialty for testing after fellowship training, with the expectation that 50% of cases will be within that field. Available subspecialties are hand, spine, pediatrics, sports, adult reconstruction, foot and ankle, trauma, and oncology. By doing so, candidates will be examined by three sets of examiners (two in each group) with at least one examiner in each group a subspecialist in the designated area [10].

Timeline

Timeline of Events Based on the 2018 Examination [4]

- April 1, 2017: 6-month case collection and applications available online.
- May & June, 2017: Must enroll patients preoperatively or perioperatively with their email addresses, for the collection of patient-reported outcomes.
- October 31, 2017: Deadline for completed application, fee, and 6-month case list.
- February 10, 2018: Deadline to submit additional documents to Credentials Committee if requested.
- April 2018: Letters of admission to examination become available on website for candidates. Candidates allowed to sit for examination have their selected cases posted online.
- June 1, 2018: Deadline to upload images and other records into the Scribe system for selected cases and pay the examination fee.
- July 24–26, 2016: Part II examinations at the Palmer House, Chicago.
- Late August, 2018: Examination results posted online for candidates.

Overview of Rules [4]

- While a candidate must have completed a residency under the rules that existed at the time residency began, candidates must meet all other requirements in effect at the time of application to sit for certification. *Candidates should check the current rules and processes at abos.org.*
- Part I must be completed before Part II. After passing the written examination, candidates have 5 years to take (and if necessary, retake) and pass the Part II oral examination. If Part II is not passed within those 5 years, which does not include time in fellowship, then retaking and passing the written examination is required before being eligible for Part II.
- Twenty months of continuous and active engagement in the practice of orthopedic surgery in one location in the United States, its territories, Canada, or a US

service installation is required. Fellowship time specifically does not count towards this 20-month period.

To sit for the oral examination in the summer of 2018, for example, the absolute latest that one could start practice would be November 1, 2016. One should consider starting no later than October 1, or even mid-September, to leave a buffer for onboarding time and not risk having to wait another year. This rule could also pose problems for those with employed positions, locum tenens, or any change in practice location within the first two years of practice.

- The application to sit for examination must be completed and credentialing accepted and the candidate admitted to the examination.
- Candidates must have a full and unrestricted license to practice medicine in the United States or Canada, or be in full-time practice in the federal government.
- While the minimum number of cases is 35 during the 6-month collection period, in a study of case mix for Part II between 1999 and 2003, candidates averaged between 117 and 129 cases, with between 15 and 17 reported complications [3].
- Candidates must collect all operative cases from all hospitals and/or surgery centers where she or he was the primary operating surgeon, including same-day surgeries, beginning April 1 of the year prior to examination.
- If a candidate is away from practice for 14 or more consecutive days during the collection period, for any reason, the starting period for collection is March 1.
- On examination day, if the candidate or examiner believes there is a conflict of interest then a replacement examiner can be requested.
- Although examiners focus on cases selected, they may also ask about a candidate's case list or practice, and there may not be time to cover all submitted materials or cases.

The ABOS has produced at checklist at: www.abos.org/certification-exams/part-ii.aspx

New in 2017: Patient Reported Outcomes

In several places, the Board notes its right to change rules and procedures at any time and without prior notice. This option was exercised in 2017, when applicants for Part II in 2018 found a brand new requirement to facilitate the collection of patient-reported outcomes (PRO) on patients. Applicants of this cycle are asked to prospectively request email addresses from patients having surgery in May and June and register them in advance through Scribe. Patients may refuse, and young children are excluded. Otherwise, patients receive PRO measures preoperatively (or perioperatively for urgent case) as well as postoperatively. While currently the means in which this information will be used to guide decisions for certification is unknown, the Board notes that such scores can be discussed during oral presentations. As this requirement is new in 2017, the future directions are unclear.

For the applicant, this process is eased by a web link and personalized password such that an administrative assistant or scheduler could ad in email addresses and register patients for the surveys. This is a new and additional requirement, which must be explained to patients, and only highlights the advice to plan additional time during the case collection period to stay up to date on data inputting. Certainly this requirement precludes the option to enter all one's cases into Scribe at the very end of the collection period.

What We Know About Predictors of Success and Failure in Part II

Between 2012 and 2016, 4–14% of candidates failed Part II [11]. There is sparse literature on what predicts difficulties at the examination, though authors with experience within the ABOS have provided guidance [10, 12]. In the context of lower pass rates for candidates listing spine surgery as their specialty or fellowship, a lower score regarding surgical indications contributed substantially [12]. This report noted several specific concerns by examiners during debriefing:

> … poor surgical indications for controversial diagnoses such as low back pain, aggressive surgical procedures without appropriate documentation, doing the same operation for any indication, and inability of a candidate to support his or her decision-making.

Candidates from all subspecialties can benefit from these insights.

At a single residency program with 16 Part II failures over 15 years, it was noted that those who failed Part II had lower OITE scores, lower Step I scores, less honors designation during medical school clinical rotations, and a weaker Deans letter [8]. This is similar to the predictions of failure in Part I. Though the paradigm is different in Canadian orthopedic training, higher OITE scores were correlated there with oral examination marks as well [13]. These studies suggest that while intuition might argue that multiple-choice scores would be less likely to predict oral examination marks, a foundation of medical knowledge and test taking acumen is helpful. More literature on strategies for success on Part II would be a useful addition to the literature and helpful for candidates.

The ABOS has offered five suggestions to Part II candidates [12]:

1. Be able to explain surgical indications in a scientific, thoughtful manner. If procedure relates to a controversial diagnosis, best evidence should be available to support the candidate's surgical decision.
2. Document carefully and fully decisions and justifications for selected cases. Candidates are specifically advised against answering, "I do it this way because that is what I learned in my fellowship."
3. Be prepared to support all decisions for selected cases, whether it is a decision for surgical or nonsurgical treatment.

4. Ensure that documentation and record-keeping are complete and organized for all cases.
5. Candidates should remember that examiners are there to test organizational skills, case preparation, knowledge, and decision-making in accordance with ABOS standards and start from a point of hoping for the success of every candidate.

Trends and Lessons from Candidate Case Lists

Case lists, submitted electronically since 1998, have also provided a nationwide orthopedic database of the care patterns of orthopedic surgeons who aim to sit for board certification [3]. The completeness of these lists is likely, due to records checks and strong motivation for compliance on the part of candidates. However, it is possible that candidates alter practice patterns during the surgical list collection period. In addition to its use for candidate evaluation certification, this database has been utilized for a variety of investigations.

Trends in care patterns have been assessed over time using candidate submitted lists. For example, between 1999 and 2003 the most common procedure was knee arthroscopy, with more than twice as many such cases as the next common procedure (carpal tunnel surgery) [3]. Over time a variety of trends have been noted, such as a transition from open to arthroscopic rotator cuff repair and less isolated subacromial decompressions [14], as well less superior labrum anterior to posterior (SLAP) repairs [15] and less arthroscopic meniscectomies, particularly among nonsports medicine fellowship trained candidates [16]. Candidates reporting trauma fellowships have submitted fewer acetabular fracture cases over time, dropping from an average of 10.1–5.2 between 2003 and 2015 while the number of pelvic ring injury and periarticular fracture cases has remained stable [17]. Another report showed a decreasing percentage of candidates treating femoral neck fractures, which could reflect subspecialization; for younger patients where open reduction internal fixation is indicated, the decreased numbers may also reflect avoidance of difficult cases [18]. The same report also noted increased use of total hip arthroplasty for femoral neck fractures, particularly by those who had completed arthroplasty fellowships, and a separate report noted that arthroplasty-trained candidates performed an increasing number of primary as well as complex revision knee arthroplasties over the course of a decade [19]. It is unknown whether these represent changes in the response to new data on the effectiveness of certain treatments, or active decisions by candidates to avoid potentially controversial indications or complication-prone operations during their case collection period. This concern about altering practice during case collection has been long noted [3].

The data have also been proposed as a means to provide orthopedic surgery residents and educators information on likely future practice [3]. This database has tracked the increasing percentage of candidates reporting fellowship training, rising to 90% by 2013, and a greater percentage of candidate cases are now within her or his subspecialty area [20]. In the case of orthopedic oncology, the finding that newly trained orthopedic oncologists only had 42% tumor cases over 10 years (35% in the later years) has implications for the subspecialty – both those hosting fellowships and for residents considering an orthopedic oncology career [21]. A more than four-fold rise in candidates with trauma fellowship training has also been reported, likewise with potential implications for workforce planning [17]. Knowing overall trends in the number and range of particular procedures may aid the Board in comparing an individual candidate's numbers against national averages to assess for extremes in either direction [3].

Preparing for Oral Examinations

Routine oral examination plays a smaller role in the United States educational paradigm than in many countries. While anyone sitting for Part II has succeeded against at least a dozen major standardized tests, direct oral examination may be less familiar. Approaches to case collection and presentation that lead to passing have not been systematically evaluated, although members of the ABOS leadership and others have provided advice for candidates.

During Case Collection

For each patient undergoing surgery, a thorough history and physical examination is expected to be documented. "Candidates are graded on how they collect data, how the information was interpreted, the preparation of a differential diagnosis, what was considered in determining a working diagnosis, the formulation of treatment options, the demonstration of technical skills, and the resulting outcome of the ultimate course of action" [5]. While this reflects good practice, it would seem wise to avoid overreliance on templated notes and to document one's thought process and any shared decision-making with the patient. This particularly applies to obtaining informed consent and discussing nonoperative and operative treatment options. Proper follow-up and documentation of end results or progress to date are also important for evaluation, and every reasonable effort should be made to secure patient follow-up.

Surely the clinical practice of orthopedics includes many difficult and unusual scenarios. Regardless of your practice situation, conventional wisdom suggests it is good for morale and one's practice to develop a mechanism for discussing challenging cases. This could be a case conference, indications conference, or something less formal. If such a discussion occurs, that could also be mentioned in a preoperative or operative note. The oral boards examination specifically evaluates operative indications [4, 5], so preoperative review of challenging cases with peers is very reasonable. At the very least it is an opportunity for you to hear other opinions, and hopefully avoid collective head scratching and statements of "I wish you'd asked my thoughts about this tough case beforehand" from peers when you start practice presentations in the spring.

All imaging will be reviewed, including preoperative and postoperative series. Take time to ensure that appropriate preoperative imaging has been obtained. As we can at times have little control over the quality of immediate postoperative imaging, consider saving important intraoperative C-arm imaging for fracture cases, as this is more within our control [22].

After Receiving Your List

When candidates receive their final case list in April of the examination year, there is a lot of work to be done. Notes must be complied, and imaging and other accompanying materials uploaded. The earlier these documents are collected and draft presentation slides made, the sooner one can start talking to colleagues about the cases. Multiple diplomates stressed the importance of broad case review and presentation practicing as I prepared this chapter. In particular, several commented on reaching out to colleagues beyond one's own institution; each hospital or group has certain entrenched ways of approaching particular clinical situations. By reviewing cases with people in a variety of regions and settings candidates gain a broader sense of anticipated questions and are able to refine the presentations and preparations. For anyone who is interested, perhaps particularly for candidates less able to seek multiple opinions, the Miller Review Course offers a highly rated one-day course that includes mock examinations and feedback.

Candidates should be able to reference relevant literature to defend treatment plans [5]. There is some debate in my discussions about whether specific articles themselves should be cited (at the risk of getting "into the weeds" during a very time-limited presentation), or just summarized to be able to support a specific treatment decision. Either way, given that there are just 12 cases and several months of preparation, it seems a safe course of action to re-review the relevant literature to one's case list. How specific or general one should respond to questions likely depends in part on the particular treatment decision.

Grading System

The Case Evaluation Rubric is readily available in the Rules and Procedures document online [4] and should be reviewed early by candidates. The categories are Data Gathering, Diagnosis and Interpretive Skills, Treatment Plan, Technical Skill, Outcomes, and Applied Knowledge. Each is scored from 3 (Excellent) to 0 (Unsatisfactory) with general descriptions of each being detailed for candidate and examiner review. There is also a Global Evaluation Rubric, which comprises Surgical Indications, Surgical Complications, and Ethics & Professionalism that is similarly scored and outlined. A failing mean score is less than 2.0 points [12].

During the Examination

The current detailed format for the day of examination processes will be provided. Practical wisdom that has been promulgated is to avoid getting defensive, take responsibilities for complications, and answer questions succinctly with the knowledge that some of the examiners may have written the book on the topic of discussion [22]. Have a clear concise summary of each case, which includes a discussion of the informed consent process and decision for operative vs. nonoperative treatment. It is in your interest to keep the pace moving and get through as many of the cases as possible in order to provide more material for evaluation [22]. Afterwards there is a debriefing section, followed by a widespread recommendation for celebrating having gotten through the day. You will not get results for about a month, so you might as well celebrate!

Resources for Part II

ABOS Website

The ABOS website is the go-to resource, and is the site you will be spending a lot of time on:

- There are recorded videos available online about Part II and using Scribe. You will also receive emails in February/March about free live webinars.

  https://abos.org/certification-exams/part-ii/videos-to-help-prepare-for-part-ii-application-and-examination.aspx
- Up-to-date rules and procedures.
- Statistics on the past several years' worth of examinations.

AAOS Offerings

- Webinar on Part II: Be watching your email or the AAOS Webinar website in January/February for opportunity to register for an information session. There is a fee associated. It can be watched live with a question and answer period, and is then available for registered participants for 30 days afterwards.
- General advice on taking oral examinations http://www.aaos.org/CustomTemplates/Content.aspx?id=6033

Orthopedic Trauma Association (OTA) Advice

The OTA provides advice for residents and fellows, including advice for case collection and more. Among its tips are to book flights and hotels as soon as you know your travel dates, do not check any critical luggage, among other helpful advice. This is definitely worth a read, though it is now a few years old.

- Advice for Part II – http://ota.org/media/87978/part-3-taking-the-exam.pdf

Miller Review Course

As with Part I, the team at Miller Review has an in-person course designed for Part II. Its current structure is a one-day course in which participants present three of their own cases, hear other case presentations and attend seminars. New in 2017 is the option for those anticipating being a candidate the following year to audit the course, as an opportunity to gain information on surgical indications and documentation during the case collection period, and to observe case presentations (http://millerreview.com).

Maintenance of Certification

For those now entering practice, certification is an unending process. And that is by design, though meandering the course has been to reach this point [23]. The ABOS vision is improving the quality of care and outcomes for patients, through competency standards and lifelong education of board-certified orthopedic surgeons. All certificates awarded after 1985 are valid for 10 years and are subject to satisfactory participation in the Maintenance of Certification (MOC) program. The term MOC is preferred over "recertification" to signify a continual process of updating knowledge and skills [23].

Elements of MOC

There are four specific MOC components consisting of evidence of professional standing lifelong learning and self-assessment, cognitive expertise, and performance in practice. Professional standing is evidenced by maintaining a full and unrestricted license to practice medicine, along with privileges at a hospital or ambulatory surgery center in the United States or Canada. The hospital or center itself must be accredited by an ABOS recognized accrediting body. Lifelong learning and self-assessment are one of the major aspects of MOC, in

Table 14.1 Elements of Maintenance of Certification (MOC)

Category	Requirements
Professional standing	Maintaining full unrestricted license
	Maintaining hospital/surgery center privileges
Lifelong learning and self-assessment	Orthopedics-related 120 Category 1 CME, by 3rd year in cycle
	Another 120 CME credits by end of 10-year cycle
	Of these, 20 credits each time (40 total) must be SAE
Cognitive expertise	Examination each 10 years
Performance in practice	Review of case list
	Peer review

Abbreviations: *CME* Continuing Medical Education, *SAE* Self-Assessment Examinations

accordance with the vision of the ABOS. In order to be considered participating in MOC, diplomates are required to submit 120 credits of Category 1 Orthopedic-related Continuing Medical Education (CME) that include a minimum of 20 CME credits of Self-Assessment Examinations (SAE) by the end of the third calendar year of one's 10-year certification cycle [4]. An additional 120 CME credits, of which 20 are SAE, must be submitted prior to scheduling an examination. In total, then, in a 10-year period the requirements are for 240 CME credits, 40 of which are SAE. Cognitive expertise is evidenced through the examinations that are part of ongoing certification every 10 years, in addition to the required SAE as part of CME. Performance in practice may be evaluated by review of a diplomate's case list, and a peer review process that requires responses from at least seven peers, five of whom must be diplomates of the ABOS (Table 14.1).

On the ABOS website, surgeons are designated as to whether they are "Participating in MOC." This has a very specific definition. Diplomates with recently awarded certifications or updated certifications receive the initial designation automatically. To keep this designation, the above required 120 CME credits must be submitted by the end of the diplomate's third calendar year of the certification cycle. If this is not done, the website designation will change to "Participating in MOC: No" until the required CME is submitted [4].

MOC Once-a-Decade Examination

There are two main options for examination at the 10-year mark. The first option is to once again submit a 6-month case list, and apply for an oral examination similar to Part II of the initial certification. This pathway may be appealing for those who work in a focused domain and have little interest in taking a computer-based examination covering topics far removed from his or her clinical practice. There are also situations in which the ABOS may require a diplomate to recertify via an oral examination pathway, which occurs if peer review has identified questions about a diplomate's practice or if there has been a limitation of surgical staff privileges by a hospital.

More commonly, though, a nonoral examination pathway is chosen by diplomates [4]. There remains a requirement to enter cases into Scribe, but only for a consecutive 3-month period or up to 75 consecutive cases performed, and these case lists do not lead to a case-based examination. Diplomates then take either a General Clinical Computer Examination or a Practice-Profiled Computer Examination. These range between 150 and 175 questions and are taken at a Prometric Center just like Part I, but are only 3 h in length. These tests are criterion-references, which means that all diplomates may pass; there is no set or minimum percentage of test takers that must fail. In addition to the general examination, there are currently seven practice-profiled computer examinations: Adult Reconstruction, Foot and Ankle, Pediatrics, Hand, Spine, Sports Medicine, and Trauma.

Can certification be removed? It absolutely can, and all diplomates are urged to read the entire rules and procedures online for additional information [4]. In addition to failure to comply with the terms and condition of the MOC process, disciplinary action by medical licensing authorities or any felony or "misdemeanor involving moral turpitude" conviction deemed by the Board to have a material relationship to the practice of medicine may result in revocation of certification.

Conclusions

The pathway to Board Certification in Orthopedic Surgery, as developed and periodically updated by the ABOS, should be a point of pride for the profession. Compared with many other specialties, or systems of orthopedic certification I have learned about in peer countries, the US system is rationally structured and of high quality. The evaluation of medical knowledge at the end of residency, combined with review of candidates' own cases in independent practice through an oral examination by established peers, is a comprehensive means of assessing competency. Of course, for those going through the process it is a significant undertaking that is both time-consuming and stressful. Hopefully the information in this chapter sheds some light on the process and provides useful information for candidates. While I have no special knowledge of the process, this chapter was put together in the midst of my own candidacy for Part II – so in the least, I was equally motivated to gather and learn what I could. I am thankful to the many people, applicants and diplomates who leant their experience and opinions on this topic. Finally, among the most important lessons for me was how the rules and processes have changed over time, even in the past few years. Candidates for certification and those in MOC should keep apprised of the current procedures through the ABOS website. Best of luck!

Terminology

- *Board certified*: an orthopedic surgeon currently certified by the ABOS.
- *Board eligible*: an orthopedic surgeon who has passed the Part I examination and is eligible to apply for completing the Part II examination for certification. This status is lost after 5 years if the oral examination is not passed.
- *Candidate*: an orthopedic surgeon applying for board certification.
- *Diplomat***e**: an orthopedic surgeon currently certified by the ABOS.
- *Maintenance of Certification (MOC):* the process through which diplomates maintain primary certification in orthopedic surgery and are assured for continuing competency.
- *Scribe*: an online program through abos.org where case lists are submitted.

References

1. Website: About ABOS. American Board of Orthopaedic Surgery. 2017. Available at: https://www.abos.org/about-abos.aspx. Accessed 14 May 2017.
2. Gundle KR. Rearticulations of orthopaedic surgery: the process of specialty boundary formation and the provision of fracture care. Online: Lulu.com; 2014.
3. Garrett WE, Swiontkowski MF, Weinstein JN, Callaghan J, Rosier RN, Berry DJ, et al. American Board of Orthopaedic Surgery Practice of the Orthopaedic surgeon: part-II, certification examination case mix. J Bone Joint Surg Am. 2006;88:660–7.
4. Website: rules and procedures for residency education, part I, and part II examinations – 2018. American Board of Orthopaedic Surgery 2017. Available at: https://www.abos.org/media/34453/2018_rules_and_procedures_part_i_part_ii_updated_2017_04_17_.pdf. Accessed 14 May 2017.
5. DeRosa GP. Topics in training: how to pass the American Board of Orthopaedic Surgery certifying examinations. J Bone Joint Surg Am. 2002;84-A(12):2309–11.
6. Website: how written examinations are developed. American Board of Orthopaedic Surgery. 2017. Available at: https://www.abos.org/certification-exams/part-i/how-written-examinations-are-developed.aspx. Accessed 14 May 2017.
7. Website: part I examination statistics. American Board of Orthopaedic Surgery. 2017. Available at: https://www.abos.org/certification-exams/part-i/exam-statistics.aspx. Accessed 14 May 2017.
8. Herndon J, Allan B, Dyer G, Jawa A, Zurakowski D. Predictors of success on the American Board of Orthopaedic Surgery Examination. Clin Orthop Relat Res. 2009;467:2436–45.
9. Dougherty P, Walter N, Schilling P, Najibi S, Herkowitz H. Do scores of the USMLE step 1 and OITE correlate with the ABOS part I certifying examination?: a multicenter study. Clin Orthop Relat Res. 2010;468:2797–802.
10. Herkowitz HN, Weinstein JN, Callaghan JJ, DeRosa GP. Spine fellowship education and its association with the part-II oral certification examination. Spine. 2006;31(20):2278–80.
11. Website: part II examination statistics. American Board of Orthopaedic Surgery. 2017. Available at: https://www.abos.org/certification-exams/part-ii/exam-statistics.aspx. Accessed 14 May 2017.
12. Herkowitz H, Emery S, Hurwitz S, Harrast J. Performance of candidates selecting the subspecialty of spine surgery for the part II American Board of Orthopaedic Surgery Oral Certification Examination. J Bone Joint Surg Am. 2013;95:e135.

13. Yen D, Athwal G, Cole G. The historic predictive value of Canadian orthopedic surgery residents' orthopedic in-training examination scores on their success on the RCPSC certification examination. Can J Surg. 2014;57:260–2.
14. Mauro C, Jordan S, Irrgang J, Harner C. Practice patterns for subacromial decompression and rotator cuff repair: an analysis of the American Board of Orthopaedic Surgery database. J Bone Joint Surg Am. 2012;94:1492–9.
15. Patterson B, Creighton R, Spang J, Roberson J, Kamath G. Surgical trends in the treatment of superior labrum anterior and posterior lesions of the shoulder. Am J Sports Med. 2014;42:1904–10.
16. Parker B, Hurwitz S, Spang J, Creighton R, Kamath G. Surgical trends in the treatment of meniscal tears. Am J Sports Med. 2016;44:1717–23.
17. Gire J, Gardner M, Harris A, Bishop J. Are early career orthopaedic trauma surgeons performing less complex trauma surgery? J Orthop Trauma. 2016;30:525–9.
18. Miller B, Callaghan J, Cram P, Karam M, Marsh J, Noiseux N. Changing trends in the treatment of femoral neck fractures. J Bone Joint Surg Am. 2014;96:e149.
19. Pour A, Bradbury T, Horst P, Harrast J, Erens G, Roberson J. Trends in primary and revision knee arthroplasty among orthopaedic surgeons who take the American Board of Orthopedics part II exam. Int Orthop. 2016;40:2061–7.
20. Horst P, Choo K, Bharucha N, Vail T. Graduates of orthopaedic residency training are increasingly subspecialized: a review of the American Board of Orthopaedic Surgery Part II database. J Bone Joint Surg Am. 2015;97(10):869–75.
21. Duchman K, Miller B. Are recently trained tumor fellows performing less tumor surgery? An analysis of 10 years of the ABOS part II database. Clin Orthop Relat Res. 2016;475:221–8.
22. Website: taking part II examination of the American Board of Orthopaedic Surgery. Banerjee R. 2009. Available at: www.ota.org/media/part-3-taking-the-exam.pdf. Accessed 14 May 2017.
23. DeRosa GP. Recertification: history of ABOS efforts. Clin Orthop Relat Res. 2006;449:149–54.

Chapter 15
Principles of Clinical Research

Richard N. Puzzitiello, Avinesh Agarwalla, Brian Forsythe, and Natalie L. Leong

What Is Clinical Research?

In the clinical or surgical setting, healthcare professionals strive to make decisions about patient care based on reported evidence. This evidence comes in the form of results from research studies that are published in medical literature journals. Clinical research uses human subjects to test the safety, efficacy, and at times superiority, of novel or pre-existing diagnostic tools, medication, devices, surgical approaches, and treatment regimens. Before reaching a clinical setting, the subject matter should be well substantiated by preclinical research of basic sciences such as physiology, pathophysiology, molecular and cellular biology, and animal research. At its core, clinical research has a bidirectional modality in that it translates basic research into medical care, and it can drive basic science research. Clinical research encompasses several types of studies, such as retrospective outcome studies, population research, and clinical trials.

When conducting research with patients, it is important to differentiate between an intervention and interaction. As defined by the Department of Health and Human Services (DHHS), an intervention includes both physical procedures (i.e., magnetic resonance imaging) and manipulations of the patient that leads to data collection. An interaction refers to the interpersonal contact, such as a survey or interview, between the investigator and subject.

Physiological research is aimed at understanding basic physiologic mechanisms in normal subjects and how those processes are disrupted in patients with a pathology. Basic science research will identify and analyze these physiologic mechanisms

R. N. Puzzitiello · A. Agarwalla · B. Forsythe · N. L. Leong (✉)
Rush University Medical Center, Midwest Orthopedics at Rush, Chicago, IL, USA

Rush University Medical Center, Department of Orthopedic Surgery, Chicago, IL, USA
e-mail: forsythe.research@rushortho.com; brian.forsythe@rushortho.com; natalie_l_leong@rush.edu

E. C. Makhni et al. (eds.), *Orthopedic Practice Management*,
https://doi.org/10.1007/978-3-319-96938-1_15

using in vitro or animal models, the results of which can be used to conduct physiologic research to confirm the presence and functionality of these pathways in human subjects. This has the capability to inform researchers of scientifically targeted medical therapy. Thus, physiologic research will inform and help direct future clinical trials. For example, physiologic research helped identify the calcium regulation pathway in humans and how that cycle is altered in various diseases processes, such as hyperparathyroidism and postmenopause. This helped drive clinical trials to determine the efficacy of drugs, such as bisphosphonates, calcitonin, and monoclonal antibodies toward rank ligand in regulating calcium levels in these disease processes.

Population research encompasses epidemiologic and behavioral research to identify high-risk patients who may benefit from prevention, early detection, or intervention of a previously acquired disease process. For example, prevention of HIV with patient education of barrier contraception, needle exchange programs, screening of HIV in sexually active patients, and early intervention of prophylactic antibiotics to reduce the incidence of opportunistic infections, has shown to reduce the prevalence of HIV and its associated complications in high-risk and general population [1–4].

Types of Clinical Research

The various types of research studies can be divided into two main categories: observational and interventional studies (Fig. 15.1). Observational studies are further categorized as prospective or retrospective, based on whether the study is designed before the intervention or data collection.

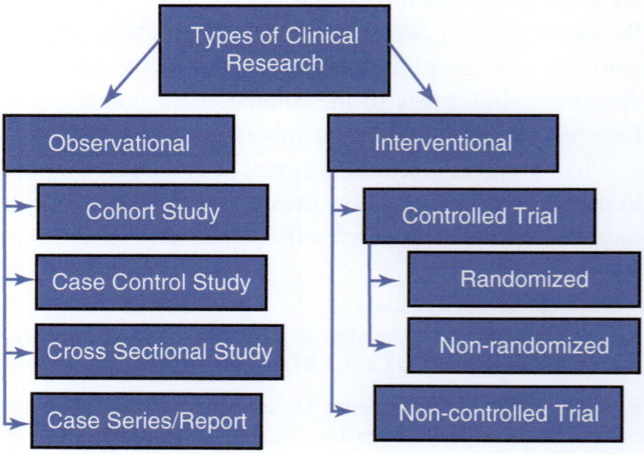

Fig. 15.1 Schematic highlighting different types of research

Case Reports/Case Series

The purpose of a case report is to document a solitary clinical observation, typically outlining the diagnosis, management, or clinical course of a patient. A case report is often utilized to illustrate a complicated or atypical patient vignette. The purpose served by a case report may be to explain a unique syndrome, abnormal disease associations, previously undocumented side effects to treatments, or a new surgical approach for a known pathology. Regardless of the content in a case report, it is still considered the lowest level of clinical evidence besides expert opinions, as they are typically reporting an exception and not the rule. Even if a case report were to document a more common clinical picture, a sample size of one would not have the power to support any speculation or conclusion. The basic utility of case reports is to present a scenario that is considered important to be documented for physicians to be aware of, but not to guide everyday clinical decision-making. Likewise, case series are reports of a small number of cases with a similar clinical scenario but are still insufficient to support any scientifically rigorous conclusions.

Case-Control Studies

Case-control studies are another type of observational study that studies a population with a disease and compares them against a similar control population without that disease. A specific exposure or risk factor is then identified to determine if there exists an association with the disease being studied. The purpose of this type of study is to retrospectively look at populations and ask, "what happened?" For example, in a study attempting to show if those who participate in competitive sports are more prone to ACL injuries, a group with ACL injuries would be compared to a control group without ACL injuries. Individuals in both groups may have the risk of participating in competitive sports, but the hypothesis would be that a larger proportion of those with ACL injuries would have this risk factor compared to the control group. This would allow for the calculation of an odds ratio, which will be further addressed in the Statistics section of this chapter.

This type of study may only suggest an association of a risk factor with a disease, but it may not prove definitively that this association is valid. This is due to the facts that other confounding variables may be present more frequently in a group that distorts the effect of risk factor on an outcome, and that the presence and timing of exposure of a risk factor may be difficult to ascertain from study populations. For these reasons, case-control studies are still considered a low level of clinical evidence. They are frequently used as a type of epidemiologic study, however, as they are inexpensive and may be less labor intensive than more structured experimental studies. The results of case-controls are effective in that they may lead to discoveries which form the basis of future clinical studies.

Cohort Studies

A cohort study is an observational study that also investigates potential risk factors or causes of a condition. The advantage of a cohort study over a case-control study is that it may be prospective or retrospective in nature. This type of study asks the question, "who will develop a disease" or "who developed a disease." A group is identified with a common risk factor or exposure at the onset, and examined over time to determine if this exposure or risk factor affects the likelihood of developing a disease. The statistical outcome measure obtained from this type of study is the relative risk, which will be discussed in further detail in the Statistics section of this chapter.

A prospectively designed cohort study has many advantages that aid in establishing causality between risk factors and an outcome. One major advantage is that the study can be highly structured from the onset, in terms of specific history or examinations taken at regular intervals, allowing for better isolation of a risk factor, or at the least allowing for better identification of confounding factors. Additionally, recall bias is reduced, which will be addressed further in a later section. For these reasons, prospective cohort studies are widely recognized as the most reliable type of observational study.

Cross-Sectional Studies

Cross-sectional studies are observational studies and are similar to cohort studies in that they analyze an exposure and an outcome; however, in a cross-sectional study, all the measurements are made at one time point with no additional follow-up. In other words, a cross-sectional study looks at a population and asks, "what is happening at only this moment." Cross-sectional studies can identify the prevalence of a condition and can describe an association between an exposure and outcome; however, a causal relationship cannot be described in this study.

Experimental Studies

An experimental study fundamentally differs from observational study in that an investigator directly administers an intervention and assesses the impact it has on a clinically measurable outcome. In doing so, the investigator is able to control who receives an exposure and who does not. Inclusion and exclusion can be set in order to define eligibility for study enrollment, thus making the population of subjects more similar. An experimental study typically contains a control group that does not receive the intervention being studied, which serves as a comparator group to asses for effect size. Outcomes are then measured in terms of absolute risk reduction (ARR), relative risk reduction (RRR), and the number needed to treat (NNT) (Table 15.1). An interventional study could possibly lack a control or comparison group, but these studies rely on extrapolations by comparing to historical control

Table 15.1 Defining terms that can describe experimental studies

Experimental studies definitions		
Term	Definition	Formula
Absolute risk reduction	Change in risk of an outcome from an intervention to a comparison treatment	$ARR = Risk_{intervention} - Risk_{comparison}$
Relative risk reduction	Determines how much an intervention reduced the risk of a bad outcome	RRR = 1 − Relative Risk
Number needed to treat	Number of people who need to be treated in order for a benefit to be seen from the intervention	$NNT = \frac{1}{ARR}$

Table 15.2 Phases and characteristics of a clinical trial

Phases of a clinical trial		
Phase	Number of patients	Goal
I	20–80	Evaluate safety, potential side effects, and appropriate dosage
II	100–130	Evaluate effectiveness of drug
III	1000–3000	Confirm effectiveness of the intervention, monitor side effects, and compare treatment to other modalities
IV	3000+	Post-market surveillance for additional risks, benefits, and maximize effectiveness

groups, implicit noninterventional outcomes, or before-after intragroup comparisons. As such, a noncontrolled study may be considered less robust and may not yield informative results.

Experimental studies are able to further reduce the possibility of reaching an inaccurate conclusion by randomizing and blinding the study. Randomization is achieved by allocating a patient who meets inclusion and exclusion criteria to either the experimental or control group randomly without knowledge of any patient information. This can be achieved by computer programs or simple random number generators. The experiment can then be single or double blinded, by preventing the patient and/or the investigator of whether the subject was randomized into the experimental or control group. A placebo is typically employed to assist in blinding. These aspects, when carried out correctly, minimize confounding effects and other types of bias, thus helping to further prove causation.

Clinical trials that are testing the therapeutic effects of a new treatment are carried out in four phases. A phase I trial is the test of the intervention on a small group of people (20–80 subjects) to evaluate its safety, potential side effects, and appropriate dosage. Phase II trials give the intervention to a larger group of people (100–300 subjects) to evaluate the effectiveness of the intervention. Phase III trials are given to an even larger group of people (1000–3000 subjects) to confirm the effectiveness of the intervention, monitor side effects, and compare the treatment modality to other treatments. Lastly, a phase IV trial includes post-marketing surveillance to determine additional risks, benefits, and how to maximize the use of the intervention (Table 15.2). Each progressing step evaluates the safety and effectiveness of a given intervention on a larger scale.

In the context of surgery, it is very difficult to design high-level studies that can aid in proving causation. For surgeries that are clearly beneficial and potentially lifesaving, it would be unethical to perform randomization and not operate on a control group. Additionally, it is impossible to double blind a surgical procedure, as the surgeon will be aware of the intervention administered. Furthermore, if two safe surgical procedures are being compared to assess for difference in outcomes, the intervention could differ within a group by the expertise of the surgeon, technique used, assistance, surgical setting, etc., which can all potentially confound the outcome. Aside from the difficulties of basic study design, individual surgeries are far less common of an intervention than medication usage, which makes it difficult to enroll a sufficient number of subjects in a reasonable timeframe. A smaller sample size then demands a higher measurable difference between groups in order to conclude an actual difference between groups. Despite the limitations on surgical research, there are methods of producing more powerful and convincing outcomes, some of which are discussed in the following section.

Systematic Reviews and Meta-Analyses

An inherent challenge that comes with conducting clinical research is controlling bias and confounding factors. These inevitable study flaws decrease reliability and present a major limitation on study results. For instance, a selected study population only represents a small fraction of the entire population, and this patient population may all share a common factor or pathology, not represented in the population as a whole. As such, the results of a research study on this population may not be reproducible in another practitioner's patient population. The purpose of a systematic review is to identify, synthesize, and appraise all the highest quality research evidence answering a common question. In the process, this identifies and minimizes the bias of each individual study. By synthesizing the data from several studies compromising numerous sample populations, the power of these studies is effectively increased. This decreases the chance of error and allows for a clearer illustration of true effect. For these reasons, comprehensive systematic reviews are at the top of the hierarchy of evidence-based medicine (Fig. 15.2).

The question being answered by a systematic review is one that is underreported, and one which identifies findings that are unique from prior reviews. The PICOS criteria describe the criterion in which studies are included and excluded in a systematic review and include the participant, intervention, comparison, outcome, and study design. Primary study outcomes are established during the study design to identify success or failure of interventions, which defines the answer to the specific question being asked. These primary outcomes are continuous with the clinical trials constituting the review. Just as with any other research study, a hypothesis regarding the study question is made prior to completing study selection as well.

Systematic reviews require the person conducting the review of the literature to be transparent in their selection process for studies to be included, so that it is clear

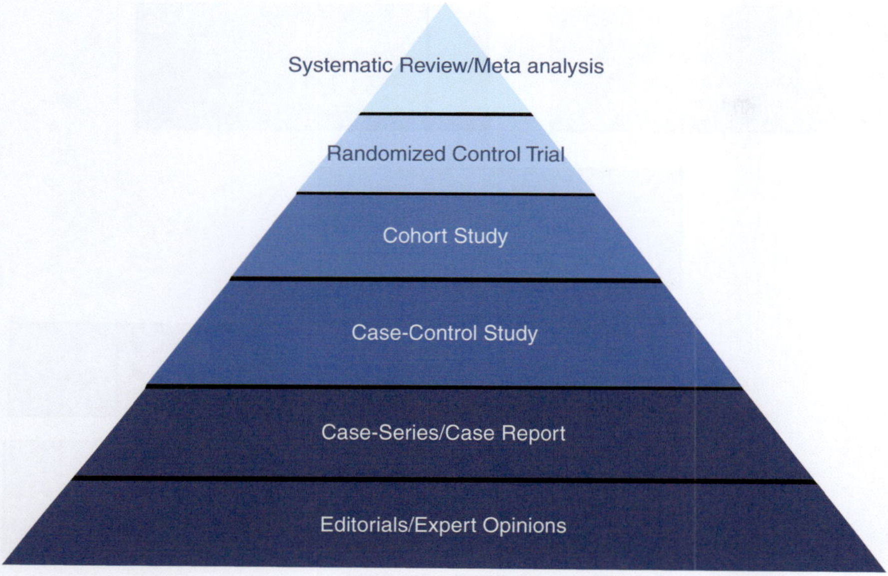
Systematic Review/Meta analysis
Randomized Control Trial
Cohort Study
Case-Control Study
Case-Series/Case Report
Editorials/Expert Opinions

Fig. 15.2 Pyramid model that stratifies the impact of various types of research modalities

that what is being reported is a comprehensive picture of the available evidence. This ensures to the reader that further bias is not being introduced by the review. A PRISMA flowchart is typically employed to document transparency in the selection process (Fig. 15.3). The studies that are selected to be included fit inclusion and exclusion criteria defined by the researches conducting the review. Loose criteria increase the sensitivity of the selection process which increases the number of potential studies (and patients) included in the review. However, this comes at the expense of increased heterogeneity in PICOS criteria. Stricter criteria may not generate enough studies and population data to answer the study question effectively. For this reason, criteria may evolve as the selection process progresses to alter the scope as the available literature demands.

There are several free electronic databases that exist that are utilized for identifying relevant studies for reviews. These databases are nonmutually exclusive, and thus duplicates can be identified among them. A systematic review is only as strong as the lowest level of evidence paper included, but a study should not be excluded only for being a low level of evidence. It is important, however, for the level of evidence of the review to be graded and reported using assessment tools such as SORT (strength of recommendation taxonomy) [5] and AMSTAR (assessment of multiple systematic reviews) [6].

After the studies meeting the set inclusion and exclusion criteria are identified, data from these studies are be extracted and analyzed. The data being extracted differ based on the question being asked and the type of studies included. Some key data that are typically extracted include publication information, study design, purposes

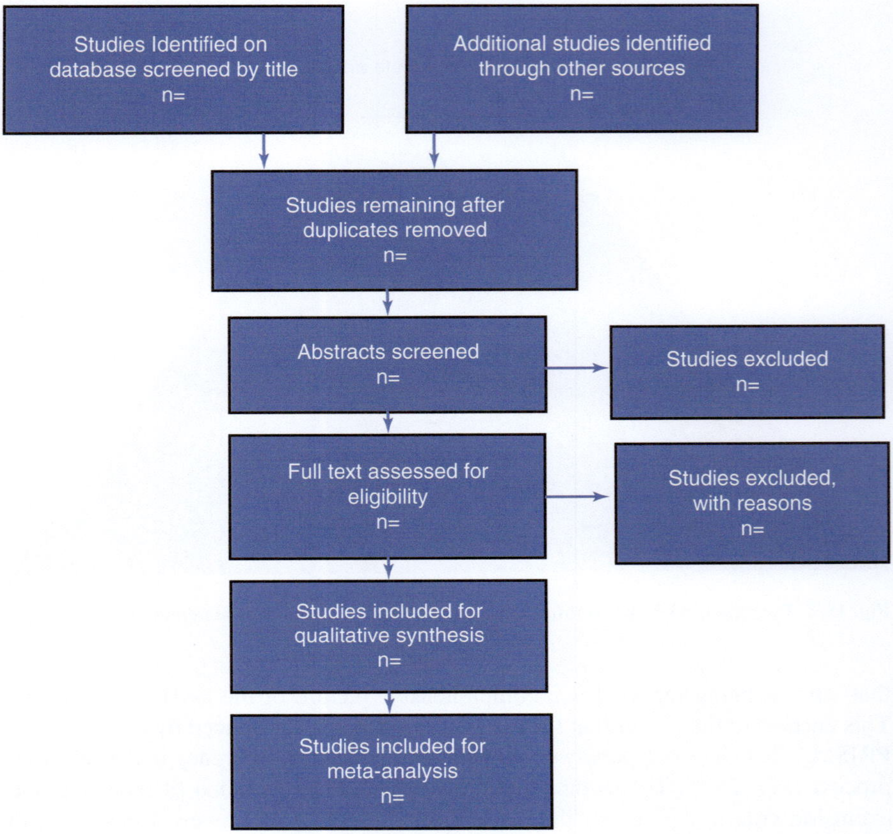

Fig. 15.3 PRISMA flowchart that is used to select articles for inclusion of a systematic review

of the study, hypotheses, outcome measures, patient criteria, intervention descriptions, comparators, and results. Once extraction is complete, similar studies with consistent interventions and outcome measures can have their results assimilated for qualitative or quantitative synthesis via meta-analysis. This may not be possible, however, due to heterogeneity among studies. Meta-analysis provides a quantitative evaluation across several sample populations. A meta-analysis needs not be comprehensive of all relevant studies included in the review, and thus subgroups can be identified and analyzed separately from the rest of the included studies to increase homogeneity in a meta-analysis. Caution should be taken when performing a meta-analysis on studies with lower evidence studies, however, as the patients may be dissimilar across study groups due to lack of randomization. A pooled analysis of lower evidence studies may help increase the number of data points, but also runs the risk of introducing new bias.

The final and most important part of a systematic review is the summary of the findings, which is presented as a final "take-home point." This statement addresses the question being asked by the review and either confirms or denies the hypothesis. The conclusion made should be substantiated by the review and analysis results. This is also when the limitations of the included studies are addressed, as these are also limitations and bias of the review. A well-conducted systematic review is revered as the gold standard in the hierarchy of evidence-based medicine, and the take-home point may be the only portion read or remembered by busy clinicians. As such, the importance of this conclusion cannot be understated.

Levels of Evidence in Clinical Research

Therapeutic

When appraising studies found in medical literature, or when submitting completed studies to journals, it is important to recognize what level of evidence the study in question is. Evidence level is a ranking system that helps grade the strength and reliability of results that are reported in research studies. The most important factor influencing level of evidence is the study design. This hierarchical system is the basis of evidence-based medicine (EBM) and should guide healthcare providers in their search for answers to clinically related questions.

Several journals and organizations have published different versions of classification schemes for different types of research questions. Therapeutic studies are often divided into five levels of evidence with levels 1–3 having subclassifications. Experimental studies are higher than observational studies in the evidence hierarchy, with systematic reviews being at the top of each level. Observational studies are ranked with cohort studies being the highest level of evidence, followed by case-control studies, then case series studies, and finally expert opinions based on principles or nonclinical studies. A study may fall into a lower level of evidence if it is poorly designed, such as if an experimental study is not randomized, or if a study is impacted by significant bias. A typical breakdown of the levels of evidence for therapeutic studies is reported in Table 15.3.

Diagnostic

In clinical studies that ask questions about diagnosis, randomized control study designs are not possible, as no intervention is being administered. The highest level of evidence in such studies is typically cohort examinations that validate a diagnostic method to a reference standard. Studies that have such convincing results that they define a positive or negative result as an absolute rule-in or rule-out of a diagnosis also have significant utility in creating a diagnostic process, and are the next highest level of evidence. At the bottom of the diagnostic study hierarchy of

Table 15.3 Studies stratified by the level of evidence

Types of studies		
	Therapeutic studies	Diagnostic studies
Level I	1. Randomized control trial 2. Systematic review of homogenous level I RCT	1. Testing of previously developed diagnostic criteria in series of patients 2. Systematic review of level I studies
Level II	1. Prospective cohort study 2. Poor-quality RCT 3. Systematic review of level II and nonhomogenous level I studies	1. Development of diagnostic criteria on consecutive patients 2. Systematic review of level II studies
Level III	1. Case-control study 2. Retrospective cohort study 3. Systematic review of level III studies	1. Study of nonconsecutive patients 2. Systematic review of level III studies
Level IV	Case series	Case-control study
Level V	Expert opinion	Expert opinion

evidence are studies that do not utilize a reference standard diagnosis as a control, retrospective case-controls, and expert opinions.

General Considerations in Clinical Research

History of Regulatory Guidelines in Human Research

In 1974, the National Research Act was formulated by the United States in order to identify basic ethical principles and develop guidelines to conduct human research. The National Research act led to 45.CFR 46 of the Department of Health and Human Services (DHHS), which defined research as "a systematic investigation, including research development, testing, and evaluation, designed to develop or contribute to generalizable knowledge." This definition of research applies broadly to studies that extend into the realm of basic sciences, such as biochemistry and biomechanics, to projects that encompass clinical questions that improve healthcare. Clinical research, as defined by the National Institutes of Health (NIH), is "research conducted with human subjects for which an investigator directly interacts with human subjects." Included in this definition of clinical research are studies that examine the effectiveness of an intervention, as well as epidemiological studies, behavioral studies, and health services. research. Clinical research is aimed at understanding human disease and improving human health. The interdependence of basic science research and clinical research (Fig. 15.4) has led to improved clinical outcomes in a myriad of diseases. For example, in the 1970s, basic science studies showed that Tamoxifen had an antitumor effect on animals. A few years later, a clinical trial demonstrated that Tamoxifen shrank breast tumors in late-stage breast cancer [7].

The act of research can often get blurred with other practices in the health field, such as innovative practice and quality assurance. While research is an investigation

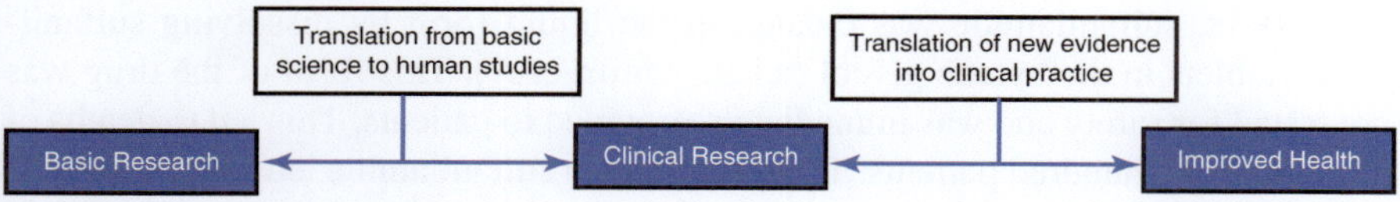

Fig. 15.4 The interdependence of clinical research and basic science research helps improve patient health and outcomes

to contribute to a pre-existing knowledge base, innovative clinical practice is an intervention designed to specifically enhance the well-being of a particular patient. Within innovative practice, an intervention is not being investigated nor is data being collected, rather a treatment is designed by a physician for the particular characteristics of a patient's case. Quality assurance projects are designed to focus primarily on enhancing patient care. within a particular environment. These projects analyze how the hospital system, ranging from physicians to ancillary staff, treat patients and how the patient's environment is affecting his or her care. The goal of a quality assurance project is to improve the patient experience in the healthcare system. These projects can improve health outcomes; however, the disadvantage of a quality assurance project is that the results of these projects are not generalizable to other patient environments.

Today, human research. has many regulations and regulatory bodies that protect the rights and well-being of human subjects. These regulations were not always in existence and have led to several ethical controversies on a national and international scale over the years that have directly led to the formation of regulatory agencies.

The Tuskegee syphilis experiment was one of the first documented examples of unethical human trials. In 1932, the US Public Health Service conducted a study to observe the progression of untreated syphilis in African American men. Researchers led subjects to believe that they were getting free healthcare from the US government; whereas in reality, these subjects received no healthcare. The study enrolled several hundred patients, many of whom developed syphilis prior to the onset of the study or during the study, but they were never told that they had the disease, nor were they treated with penicillin – even after the drug was shown to be effective in treating syphilis. This study led to numerous men who died of syphilis, women who contracted the disease from their partners, as well as many children who developed congenital syphilis.

This study directly led to the Belmont Report in 1979 which summarizes ethical principles and guidelines for research in human. subjects. The Belmont Report is comprised of three principles: respect for persons, beneficence, and justice. Respect for persons ensures that patients are treated as autonomous people and not as an asset. Beneficence states that design for a research project should be formulated to maximize benefit and minimize harm. Lastly, justice ensures that all people be treated fairly and equitably. The Tuskegee syphilis experiment also led to establishment of the Office for Human Research Protections (OHRP) – which functions to regulate the Institutional Review Boards.

In 1938, sulfanilamide was created in the liquid form by dissolving sulfanilamide tablets in diethylene glycol (a.k.a. "antifreeze"). This form of the drug was not tested for safety and was immediately provided to patients. This led to deaths of more than one hundred patients. The disaster with sulfanilamide led to formation of the US Food, Drug, and Safety Act which requires drug manufacturers to ensure drug safety as well as efficacy through extensive preclinical and clinical research testing, prior to releasing the drug for clinical use [8].

During World War II, the Germans conducted many studies. on humans without consent or any previous foundational studies to guide their work. Many studies resulted in the torture and death of prisoners in concentration camps. As a result of these actions, the Nuremberg Code was created in 1947 to help provide structure to human research. The Nuremberg Code calls for research where the risks are weighed against the benefits, physical and mental suffering is avoided, and where death or severe injury is not an expected outcome. The code also calls for the need for informed consent and protocols based on prior animal studies. Although this list was paramount in providing structure to human research, it had very little impact in the United States, as it was viewed as a mechanism to condemn Nazis rather than a code for human research worldwide. Additionally, there was no law enforcement agency to uphold the code.

The limitations of the Nuremberg Code led to formulation of the Declaration of Helsinki in 1964. The Declaration of Helsinki was created by the World Medical Association (now known as World Health Organization), and it created a code of ethics geared toward therapeutic medical research that had a broader scope than the Nuremberg Code. The Declaration of Helsinki required that potential participants maintain their autonomy to make informed decisions regarding inclusion in a study prior to beginning the study and at any point during the course of the study. The Declaration ensures that investigators maintain the patient's best interest. and provide special vigilance to those who cannot give proper consent, such as minors or the mentally incompetent.

Current Regulations

Prior to the 1940s, clinical research was largely unregulated. This yielded several ethical controversies and violations, such as the Tuskegee Syphilis Experiment. Studies like these have led to the regulation of research from basic science to clinical science. Regulatory agencies ensure that those conducting experiments, animal specimens, and human subjects are treated with the utmost respect. The Food and Drug Administration regulates the approval process of drugs, supplements, and medical devices to ensure the safety, efficacy, and security of those materials. The Office of Human Research Protections (OHRP) protects the rights, welfare, and well-being of research subjects enrolled in studies that are supported by the Department of Health and Human Services. Each institution that conducts research has its own local Institutional Review Board (IRB), which conducts initial review of research proposals. An IRB typically consists of both scientists and nonscientists from diverse backgrounds, and ensures that participants in a study receive proper informed consent and are not exposed to unreasonable risks. Throughout the study, the IRB has safeguards in place that allow them to ensure that protections of human subjects remain enforced. The IRBs, in turn, report to the OHRP.

As defined by the NIH, clinical trials are research studies that examine whether a medical strategy, treatment, or device is effective and safe for use in humans. While existing treatments, medications, and devices can be studied or compared without federal regulation, novel therapies or therapeutic devices must be approved by the US Food and Drug Administration (FDA). These studies are conducted after testing has been completed in animal models and has shown evidence of safety, and are submitted to the FDA as an investigational new drug (IND) or investigational device exemption (IDE).

While what constitutes an IND may be intuitive, an IDE can be more ambiguous. A medical device is defined as something that is not intended to have any chemical action or to be metabolized. This may be something as simple as a tongue depressor or as complex as a prosthetic joint implant. While all INDs have regulatory requirements from the FDA, not all medical devices do. A medical device falls into one of three classifications, with each class device being of increasing risk. Class I devices are widely regarded as safe and are exempt from regulation. Class II and III devices require an IDE submission to the FDA before clinical testing. If the IDE is approved, then clinical trials can be conducted to collect data to support a premarket notification 510(k) (for class II devices), or a premarket approval (PMA) (for class III devices). The testing to support 510(k)s is typically performance testing showing equivalence to an existing device, and PMA testing has stricter requirements for clinical data showing assurance of safety and effectiveness. Once a PMA or 510(k) is approved, the device may be introduced to the market.

Regarding clinical trials in the context of orthopedic surgery, drugs are rarely studied, devices are studied fairly frequently, but the most common types of clinical trials are outcomes and comparisons of different surgical procedures or approaches. Surgical technique or procedure innovation requires little to no regulation, but the development of them can be equally complicated. In general, the development of new surgical procedures is guided by ethical principles such as a physicians' oath to "do no harm," and by internal institutional oversight such as by an IRB. A new procedure may be a variation of an existing theme, or a new theme altogether. For example, when first performed, using an autograft to reconstruct an ACL was a new theme, whereas when a bone-patellar tendon-bone autograft was first used, this was a variation of a theme. New themes often begin as experimental trials in animals and progress to small human trials once proven to be efficacious and safe. These small human trials are often published as case reports in journals or at conferences to be disseminated. As for variations on techniques, there is a large "gray area" of surgical innovation as to what constitutes research versus therapeutic intervention. As such, the formal systematic process of regulating surgical innovation is not nearly as regulated as the introduction of drugs and devices to the market. The introduction and refinement of new surgical advances is thus more haphazard. In this absence of regulatory guidelines, it falls on the ethical boundaries of individual surgeons and the influence of peers and institutional boards, to decide what constitutes ethical research and innovation.

Sources of Research Funding

Funding for clinical research comes from several major sources, such as the federal government, state and local government, and private organizations. As of 2016, there were more than 26 million publications in the PubMed database. As this number has continued to rise over the years, funding for research has continued to increase from various sectors. From 1994 to 2012, medical research funding has nearly doubled from $59.5 billion dollars in 1994 to $116.5 billion dollars in 2012. During this time, the largest contributors to this budget have been the pharmaceutical firms (32% in 2012) and the National Institutes of Health (27% in 2012). The NIH is the major source of funding for research via the federal government. The biotechnology industry contributes the third largest amount of resources for research, accounting for 17% of the medical research funding in 2012 [9].

Another major source of funding for research comes from the Veterans Administration (VA). Research funding from the VA is intramural, meaning that it is accessible only to scientists employed by the VA. Such research typically focuses on areas of particular clinical interest with regard to veterans.

Funding for research comes from many other sources besides the NIH and VA. Funding for clinical research from the federal government also arises from the Agency for Healthcare Research and Quality, Center for Disease Control and Prevention, and the Department of Defense, among other agencies. The private sector is also a major contributor for funding of clinical research. As discussed previously, pharmaceutical, biotechnology, and medical device firms contribute significant funds for clinical research. Also, not-for-profit organizations donate money for research on specific topics that support the goal of that organization. Lastly, much clinical research in orthopedic surgery is nonfunded or self-funded by an investigator or institution.

Challenges in Study Execution

Clinical research has significant utility in improving healthcare; however, clinical researchers face significant challenges in conducting research. Many clinical researchers conduct research in addition to fulfilling their primary role in providing patient care. Often times, finding a balance between clinic responsibilities and research interests is difficult. This can lead to studies that do not get pursued, completed, or prioritized due to other responsibilities. In order to maintain the integrity of research, many regulatory agencies require a significant amount of paperwork, which can be a deterrent for researchers in pursuing a clinical question.

A significant proportion of clinical studies are conducted at educational institutions. From a financial standpoint, researchers at academic centers have a lower earning potential than their colleagues who pursue a position in private practice. A survey conducted by the Medical Group Management Association in 2009 demonstrated that the average salary for a primary care physician at an academic institution was $158,218 annually, whereas the average salary of a primary care physician in private practice was $186,044 annually. The difference in salary may drive physicians into private practice, which decreases participation and contribution toward clinical research.

Lastly, conducting clinical research is difficult due to the low success rate of research grants. The R01 grant from the National Institute of Health provides support for health-related research and development. According to the NIH, success rate of the R01 grant in 2016 was 19.96%. This low success rate prevents a significant proportion of studies that may have significant clinical utility from getting pursued.

Implementing changes to improve the landscape of clinical research is paramount to enhancing recruitment and retention of clinical researchers. This allows for optimization of translation of bench to bedside science, which can drive further discoveries in basic science as well as improving human health. These challenges experienced by clinical researchers can potentially be mitigated by instituting several policies or improving existing protocols. For example, improved mentoring by senior clinical researchers can help younger clinical researchers understand the process of conducting efficient research, such that a clinician researcher's time can be utilized more effectively.

If regulatory requirements are standardized, the paperwork associated with initiating a study can be less burdensome, which can improve follow-through on a study. Additionally, increasing the number of clinical researchers on review panels for clinical research grants can improve success rates for grant proposal, as well as improve feedback that is provided to clinicians who do not have an initial successful grant proposal. Lastly, expanding access to loan forgiveness programs to offset the difference in earning potential between those in academia versus private practice may assist in retaining clinicians within the research realm. Regardless of the mechanism, there stands the potential to assist clinicians in conducting research to make the process less burdensome and focus primarily on understanding physiologic and pathophysiologic mechanisms to improve overall health.

Bias in Research

A crucial consideration of clinical research is research bias, which is defined as a deviation in study design that prejudices outcomes which threatens the validity of the results. Bias is what limits studies and ultimately decides what level of evidence a study represents. There is no way to eliminate every possible bias in a study design, but measures can be taken to minimize bias, such is the goal of randomization and blinding. Bias has the ability to create an apparent association or obscure results in profound ways, and it is the job of the researcher and the one appraising the evidence to identify and consider bias in attempting to answer any research question.

There are two major types of bias that occur in research – random and systematic bias. Random bias is an unavoidable phenomenon that occurs due to variations within a sample that are extrapolated to represent a larger population. This type of bias is addressed, however, by statistical analysis after a studies' completion. The other type of bias that exists is systematic bias which is a phenomenon that is reproducible and consistent flaw that affects perceived results to differ from reality. Systematic bias is addressed in the study design of clinical research.

The major categories of systematic bias include selection biases, measurement biases, and interventional biases. Selection biases can result in comparing an experimental group to a control group that is dissimilar and thus may show a different outcome that is associated with their baseline differences and not the exposure or intervention being studied. Measurement bias can occur during data collection and can occur due to inconsistent instrumentation, a subject's ability to recall, and an experimenter's expectation of seeing a certain result, among many other things. Intervention bias can be anything that affects the treatment of exposure so that it is not consistent among subjects or is altered by an unmeasured external factor.

Basic Statistics for Clinical Research

Statistics is a crucial aspect of any type of research that puts the results of studies into perspective and helps communicate outcomes in meaningful and consistent ways. There are many ways to report data, but only certain statistical calculations can be made on a specific dataset depending on the type of data being reported. Selecting the correct test and properly calculating a statistic can be a challenging test, and as such a professional statistician is often consulted when interpreting experimental results.

Types of Data

Data can either be discrete or continuous. If the measured variable falls within a particular category, it is known as discrete data. For example, a positive or negative result on a screening test or a subjects' gender or race would classify as discrete data. Discrete data measures the frequency of occurrence and statistical tests such as chi-square test can be used to analyze such results. On the other hand, continuous data represents measurement of data that can be characterized as having an infinite number of possibilities. Examples of continuous data include measurements of a subject's height and weight. Often, discrete data and continuous data can be measured together within a study. For example, patients can be stratified into groups based on decade of life (discrete data), and within those groups, subjects can be organized by weight (continuous data).

Distribution of Data

When conducting a study, it is unlikely that a treatment or intervention can be administered to the entire population of interest. Thus, investigators analyze a subset of patients, from which a conclusion can be drawn and be applied to the entire population. The subjects from the population that are used to conduct the study must be chosen in such a way that they represent the entire population of interest. For example, if an investigator wanted to analyze the effects of repeated trauma on the knee in contact sports, it is unreasonable to expect that the investigator can analyze every individual who is involved in contact sports. Thus, the investigator must analyze a subset of this population to conduct his study. It is important to note that populations are unique; however, samples of that population are not unique [10].

For a given sample of the population, the investigator will find a mean value for the variable of interest. Another investigator may select a different sample of the population and find a different mean value for the variable of interest. Statistical theory exists to account for this sample-to-sample variation [11].

A statistical sample is reported as normal or a Gaussian distribution if the samples demonstrate a symmetric, bell-shaped distribution. The definition of a normal distribution does not allow for conclusions to be drawn from the distribution. Rather a normal distribution defines the dataset as being bell-shaped with a single peak at the mean. In the same light, if a distribution is described as nonnormal, it does not indicate that the results of the data are abnormal. Instead, an abnormal distribution indicates that the sample does not have a single, symmetric peak centered at the mean, but the distribution may have a bimodal peak or a skewed distribution. When analyzing these datasets, the data must be transformed using a logarithm or square root analysis to convert the data to a normal distribution [11].

A normal distribution is the basic underlying premise for performing accurate statistical analysis. The mean and standard deviation from a sample is used to estimate the mean and standard deviation of the population. The mean represents the average of the sample and is a measure of central tendency, alongside median and mode. The standard deviation is the measure of the spread of the data. As the mean is changed, the peak of the distribution will translate horizontally along the axis. As the standard deviation changes, the breadth of the curve is altered. The smaller the standard deviation, the narrower the curve is; whereas, the larger the standard deviation is, the distribution of the variables will be spread across the axis (Fig. 15.5).

In a Gaussian distribution, the data exhibit the 68–95–99.7 rule which states that the 68% of the data will be within 1 standard deviation of the mean, while 95% of the data will be within 2 standard deviations, and 99.7% of the data will be within 3

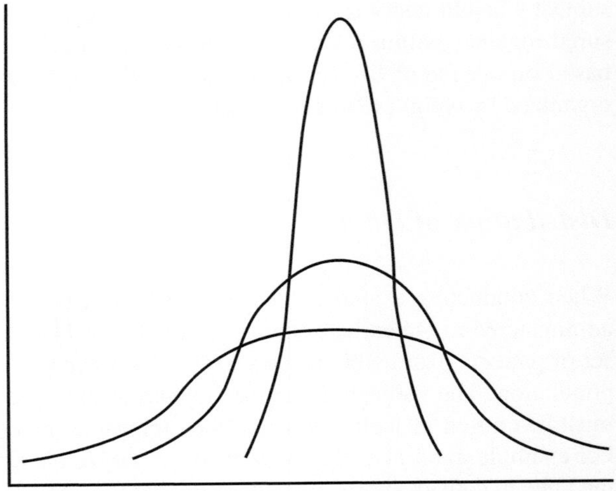

Fig. 15.5 If the variance in a population is large, the curve is wide. As the variance decreases, the narrower the curve becomes

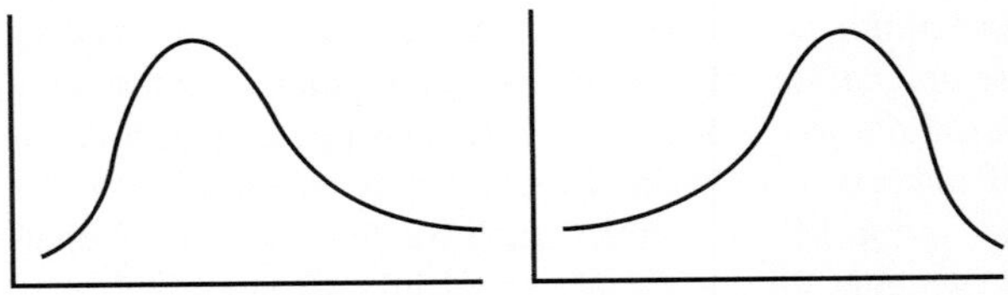

Fig. 15.6 Data that are skewed left and right. The direction of skewedness refers to the direction of the tail. LEFT: skewed right. RIGHT: skewed left

standard deviations of the mean in a normally distributed sample. In some cases, the samples may have a large proportion of data centered around some value, while there are several measurements that are significantly larger or smaller than the majority of the data. This causes the standard curve to be skewed toward the larger or smaller values (Fig. 15.6).

Measures of Central Tendency

Measures of central tendency demonstrate where data in the sample are centered along the continuance of possible values. These measures of central tendency consist of the mean, median, and mode. The mean is calculated by adding the values of all the measurements and dividing that sum by the total number of measurements. It is the most commonly used measure of central tendency. Unfortunately, the mean is subject to influence by extreme values.

Median is another measure of central tendency and it is the middle value of the dataset that is ordered from smallest to largest. If the dataset has an even number of measurements, the median is calculated by taking the average of the two middle values of the ordered dataset. The median is less sensitive to extreme values. Mode is the most frequently occurring value of the dataset. The mode must be a value that occurs more than once in the dataset. In a normally distributed dataset, the meanis equal to the median and mode.

Measures of Spread

Spread measures the variability of the sample. Consider, for example, a patient who has two readings of bicep flexion strength test of 50 foot-lbs, while another patient has two readings of bicep flexion strength test of 40 foot-lbs and 60 foot-lbs. In both cases, the mean and median are the same; however, in the latter example, there is variability in the measurements of strength. Measurements of variation include range, variance, standard deviation, and standard error.

Range the difference between the largest value and the smallest value in the dataset. A more informative measure of variation in a sample is variance. Variance is calculated by taking the difference from an individual observation from the mean and squaring that value. This is done for each measurement in the sample set, and the values are summed together. This sum is divided by the sample size minus one (n-1) (Eq. 15.1). The advantage of variance is that it incorporates all the values of a dataset; however, the main disadvantage of variance is that it is not in the same physical units as the sample set. To obtain a value that has physical meaning, the square root of the variance is obtained to get the standard deviation (Eq. 15.2). Standard deviation is the most commonly reported measure of variance.

$$\text{variance} = \frac{\Sigma\left(x_i - \bar{x}\right)^2}{n-1} \tag{15.1}$$

$$\text{St. Dev.} = \sqrt{\frac{\Sigma\left(x_i - \bar{x}\right)^2}{n-1}} \tag{15.2}$$

The final measure of variation is standard error. The standard error measures the variability from statistic to statistic as well as sample to sample. It is calculated by taking the standard deviation and dividing it by the square root of number of samples (n) (Eq. 15.3).

$$\text{St. Error} = \frac{\sqrt{\frac{\Sigma\left(x_i - \bar{x}\right)^2}{n-1}}}{\sqrt{n}} \tag{15.3}$$

Measure of Disease Frequency

Epidemiology is the study of disease frequencies in human populations [12]. Prevalence is the number of existing cases of a disease divided by the total population at a given moment in time (Eq. 15.4). For example, if there are three cases of shoulder inflammation in baseball players at the onset of the season in a population of 100 players who are at risk, the prevalence is 3%. On the other hand, incidence is the number of new cases that develop over a period of time. Incidence can be examined in two ways: cumulative incidence and incidence rate. Cumulative incidence is the number of new cases that develop over a specific time period divided by the number of people without the disease at the onset of the time period (Eq. 15.5). Returning to our example of shoulder inflammation, if 10 patients develop shoulder inflammation over the course of a season, the cumulative incidence is 10.3% since 98 players did not have shoulder inflammation at the onset of the season, whereas the prevalence at the beginning of the time period was 3% and then it was 13% at the end of the season.

$$\text{Prevalence} = \frac{\#\,\text{cases}}{\text{Total}\,\#\,\text{people}} \tag{15.4}$$

$$\text{Cumulative Incidence} = \frac{\dfrac{\#\,\text{new cases}}{\text{time}}}{\#\,\text{people without disease at onset}} \tag{15.5}$$

The downside of cumulative incidence is that it does not account for varying levels of time that a person is exposed to risk factor for an injury or illness. Therefore, it is not a precise measurement of incidence rate. Incidence rate is the number of new cases that develop during a given time period divided by the total time of exposure (Eq. 15.6). Going back to our example of shoulder inflammation, if risk for the disease is increased in starting pitchers (who pitch longer in a given game) than relievers (who may pitch only one inning in a game), cumulative incidence does not take that into account. However, incidence rate takes the population at risk as well as each person's time of risk into account by adding up the innings of exposure over the course of the season. In our example of shoulder inflammation, 10 patients developed inflammation during the season. If in the sample being tested, the pitchers collectively pitched a total of 1000 innings, the incidence rate is 10 new cases of shoulder inflammation/1000 innings pitched.

$$\text{Incidence Rate} = \frac{\#\,\text{new cases}}{\text{Total time of Exposure}} \tag{15.6}$$

Often times a relationship exists between a risk factor and development of a disease. For example, those who participate in contact sports have an increased risk of rupturing their anterior cruciate ligament (ACL). There are two ways to express this relationship: relative risk and odds ratio. Relative risk estimates the significance of the association between a risk factor and an injury. It indicates the likelihood of developing a disease in a group of subjects who are exposed to a risk factor compared to those who are not exposed to that risk factor. Relative risk is the incidence of injury/disease in those exposed to a risk factor divided by the incidence of injury/disease in those not exposed to the risk factor (Table 15.4, Eqs. 15.7 and 15.8). Equation 15.8 refers to Table 15.5 to describe its variables. To assess the risk of increased innings pitched in developing shoulder inflammation, we would check the incidence of developing inflammations in patients who are starting pitchers as well as the incidence of developing shoulder inflammation in patients who are relief pitchers. If 8 out of 50 starting pitchers develop shoulder inflammation (incidence = 16%), while 2 out of 50 relief pitchers developed shoulder inflammation (incidence = 4%), the relative risk would be the incidence in starting pitchers (16%) divided by the incidence in relief pitchers (4%) – yielding a relative risk of 4.

$$\text{Relative Risk} = \frac{\dfrac{\text{Incidence Injury}}{\text{Exposed to Risk Factor}}}{\dfrac{\text{Incidence Injury}}{\text{Unexposed to Risk Factor}}} \tag{15.7}$$

$$\text{Relative Risk} = \frac{\dfrac{a}{a+b}}{\dfrac{c}{c+d}} \tag{15.8}$$

A relative risk of 1 shows that exposure to a risk factor has no effect in developing a disease/injury. A relative risk greater than 1 indicates that exposure to a risk factor increases the likelihood of developing a disease/injury. The higher the value

Table 15.4 Calculation of relative risk and odds ratio

	Disease	
	Yes	No
Exposure		
Yes	A	b
No	C	d

Table 15.5 Actual values in chi-square test

	Disease		
Exposure	Yes	No	Total
Yes	a	b	$a + b$
No	c	d	$c + d$
Total	$a + c$	$b + d$	N

of the relative risk, the stronger the association is between the risk factor and development of disease. If the risk factor is measured on a continuous scale (i.e., innings pitched), the risk can be assessed as a function of exposure allowing for a dose-dependent relationship to be established between the exposure and outcome. A relative risk less than one indicates a protective effect of the exposed factor in developing the disease/injury. Relative risk is best assessed by a cohort study which is discussed in further detail in the next section.

Often times a study is a case-control study in which patients are selected due to the presence or absence of a disease. In these studies, investigators calculate the odds ratio. Odds ratio explores the odds of a certain exposure in those with the disease process compared to those who do not have the disease process (Eqs. 15.9, 15.10 and 15.11). Equation 15.11 references Table 15.4. For example, if a physician is asked to assess 100 patients, they fall into two categories: those with previous history of shoulder inflammation ($n = 20$) and those without a history of shoulder inflammation ($n = 80$). Of the 20 patients with a history of shoulder inflammation, 15 were starting pitchers, while 5 were relief pitchers. Of the 80 patients without a history of shoulder inflammation, 50 were relief pitchers and 30 were starting pitchers. The odds ratio is 5. This means that patients who are starting pitchers were five times more likely to get shoulder inflammation than those who were relief pitchers.

$$\text{Odds Ratio} = \frac{\text{Probability of exposure among those with disease}}{\text{Probability of exposure among those without disease}} \tag{15.9}$$

$$\text{Odds Ratio} = \frac{P\left(\frac{\text{exposed}}{\text{diseased}}\right) P\left(\frac{\text{not exposed}}{\text{not diseased}}\right)}{P\left(\frac{\text{not exposed}}{\text{diseased}}\right) P\left(\frac{\text{exposed}}{\text{not diseased}}\right)} \tag{15.10}$$

$$\text{Odds Ratio} = \frac{\dfrac{\left(\frac{a}{a+c}\right)}{\left(\frac{c}{a+c}\right)}}{\dfrac{\left(\frac{b}{b+d}\right)}{\left(\frac{d}{b+d}\right)}} = \frac{\frac{a}{c}}{\frac{b}{d}} = \frac{ad}{cb} \tag{15.11}$$

When calculating relative risk or odds ratio, a single value should not be reported, rather a range of values – confidence interval – is reported. The confidence interval provides a range at which the true relative risk or odds ratio lies. It should be noted that the odds ratio and relative risk do not indicate causality, rather it reports an association between the risk factor and disease. Lastly, if a disease has a low incidence profile, odds ratio is equal to relative risk.

The most important and commonly used statistical test is to compute a *p*-value. As will be discussed later on in this section, *p*-value is important to assessing significance of a result. If the data being evaluated are continuous and can be reported as mean values, then a student t-test or an analysis of variance (ANOVA) test can be performed to obtain the *p*-value. The student t-test is the most common modality in determining a *p*-value. In this test, the means of two groups are being compared to one another. The t-statistic is calculated by the difference between the sample mean and the hypothesized population mean divided by the standard error (Eq. 15.12). The t-statistic and the degrees of freedom (n-1) are used together to calculate the *p*-value. The means of two different groups can be compared using an unpaired t-test, or the means of a single group at two different points in time can be compared using a paired t-test. For example, if patients were enrolled in a study examining the efficacy of surgical techniques for a particular pathology, an unpaired t-test could be used to assess the difference in efficacy between the two groups at a postoperative time point. If patients were assessed preoperatively for functionality and were assessed again at 1 year postoperatively, the change in functionality among patients could be assessed using a paired t-test.

$$t^* = \frac{\bar{x} - x_o}{\frac{s}{\sqrt{n}}} \tag{15.12}$$

In the event that the study needs to examine the relationship between more than two variables, ANOVA is the test of choice. The calculation of ANOVA by hand is a lengthy process and is often deferred to a statistical package for evaluation; thus, it is out of the scope of this chapter. If the data from an experiment are percentages or proportions of categorical outcomes, then a chi-square test should be performed. In this test, the totals of each variable in the groups (total number of disease and nondisease; total number of exposure and nonexposure) are used to create the expected values for each grouping (Tables 15.5 and 15.6). These expected values and actual values are then used to calculate *p*-values alongside the degrees of freedom (n-1) (Eq. 15.13). The chi-square test is often not performed by hand, rather it is computed using a statistical software.

$$\chi_c^2 = \Sigma \frac{O_i - E_i)^2}{E_i} \tag{15.13}$$

Calculating statistics can be a difficult process that can lead to errors in calculating, reporting, and drawing of conclusions. It is advisable to consult a statistician and/or utilize statistical software.

Table 15.6 Predicted values in chi-square test

	Disease		
Exposure	Yes	No	Total
Yes	$\frac{(a+c)*(a+b)}{N}$	$\frac{(b+d)*(a+b)}{N}$	$a + b$
No	$\frac{(a+c)*(c+d)}{N}$	$\frac{(b+d)*(c+d)}{N}$	$c + d$
Total	$a + c$	$b + d$	N

Evaluation of Diagnostic Tests

There are several statistical measures used to evaluate the performance of diagnostic tests which utilize known disease prevalence and binary testing results. The two most widely utilized measures are sensitivity, or the true positive rate, and specificity, or true negative rate. Sensitivity is the proportion of individuals who actually have the disease being tested for over all individuals who tested positive for the disease. Screening tests such as a colonoscopy should have high levels of sensitivity that approach 100%, so that all individuals who have a disease will be identified by the test. These tests help rule out a disease in the target population, as there is a decreasing likelihood that they will test negative if they do not have the disease. Specificity is the proportion of individuals without a disease that tests negative. Tests that are used to confirm an initial diagnosis should have a high specificity so that there is a low rate of false positives. Sensitivity and specificity are fixed properties of diagnostic tests, and they are inversely correlated with each other; a test with a high sensitivity typically comes at the expense of the specificity of the test.

Two additional statistical measures that can be used in evaluating diagnostic tests are positive predictive value and negative predictive value. The positive predictive value of a test is defined as the proportion of positive test results in the population that actually have the disease being tested for. The negative predictive value is simply the inverse of the positive predictive value, the proportion of negative test results in the population that do not have the disease. These tests are not fixed properties of a test unlike sensitivity in specificity. Their values vary with prevalence and pretest probability. For example, in an older population of smokers, a chest CT exam will have a high positive predictive value and low negative predictive value for detecting lung cancer.

A 2 × 2 table (Table 15.7) can be constructed when disease prevalence for a population is known that can aid in calculating sensitivity (Eq. 15.14), specificity (Eq. 15.15), negative predictive value (Eq. 15.16), and positive predictive value (Eq. 15.17).

Table 15.7 Standard table used to calculate sensitivity, specificity, PPV, NPV

	Disease	
Exposure	Yes	No
Yes	True positive (TP)	False positives (FP)
No	False negatives (FN)	True negatives (TN)

$$\text{Sensitivity} = \frac{\text{TP}}{\text{TP} + \text{FN}} \tag{15.14}$$

$$\text{Specificity} = \frac{\text{TN}}{\text{TN} + \text{FP}} \tag{15.15}$$

$$\text{PPV} = \frac{\text{TP}}{\text{TP} + \text{FP}} \tag{15.16}$$

$$\text{NPV} = \frac{\text{TN}}{\text{TN} + \text{FN}} \tag{15.17}$$

Significance

Research studies report their findings as statistically significant or not, by conducting statistical analysis comparing two outcome values of the experimental and control group, yielding a *p*-value. Prior to beginning a study, investigators form a null hypothesis which states that there is no association between the variable they are investigating and the outcome. Investigators will also set a significance level, which is usually 0.05. This value denotes that there must be less than a 5% chance that the results of the study are due to chance alone. *P*-values that are less than the significance level indicate that the evidence is strong to reject the null hypothesis and conclude that there is an association between the intervention and outcome. A *p*-value greater than the significance level fails to reject the null hypothesis indicating that there is no association between the intervention and outcome. Thus, any association may be due to random chance.

Errors can occur during statistical testing with regard to assessing *p*-values and drawing conclusions. The most common types of errors are type I and type II errors. A type I error is when the null hypothesis (stating that there is no association between the intervention and outcome) is true, but it is rejected. This type of error is similar to a false positive, where researchers are associating a relationship that is absent. The error rate of a type I error is the significance level of rejecting the null hypothesis, the alpha level. In most studies, this significance level is set to 0.05 (5%). In a type II error, the null hypothesis is accepted when in reality it should be rejected. This type of error is similar to a false negative, where researchers fail to recognize a relationship that exists. The error rate of a type II error is denoted by β.

Conclusion

In summary, this chapter reviewed different types of clinical research, considerations in research such as funding sources, regulations, and challenges to performing research, as well as basic statistics. Hopefully, this overview will help the reader to better understand clinical research and possibly contribute to the growing body of orthopedic literature.

References

1. Weller SC. A meta-analysis of condom effectiveness in reducing sexually transmitted HIV. Soc Sci Med. 1993;36(12):1635–44.
2. Hurley SF, Jolley DJ, Kaldor JM. Effectiveness of needle-exchange programmes for prevention of HIV infection. Lancet. 1997;349(9068):1797–800.
3. Moyer VA. Force* USPST. Screening for HIV: U.S. preventive services task force recommendation statement. Ann Intern Med. 2013;159(1):51–60.
4. Service USPH, Infectious Diseases Society of A, Group UIPoOIW. 2001 USPHS/IDSA guidelines for the prevention of opportunistic infections in persons infected with human immunodeficiency virus. HIV Clin Trials. 2001;2(6):493–554.
5. Ebell MH, Siwek J, Weiss BD, et al. Strength of recommendation taxonomy (SORT): a patient-centered approach to grading evidence in the medical literature. J Am Board Fam Pract. 2004;17(1):59–67.
6. Shea BJ, Hamel C, Wells GA, et al. AMSTAR is a reliable and valid measurement tool to assess the methodological quality of systematic reviews. J Clin Epidemiol. 2009;62(10):1013–20.
7. Cole MP, Jones CT, Todd ID. A new anti-oestrogenic agent in late breast cancer. An early clinical appraisal of ICI46474. Br J Cancer. 1971;25(2):270–5.
8. Ballentine C. Sulfanilamide disaster. In: Administration USFaD, ed. FDA Consumer Magazine, 1981.
9. Moses H, Matheson DH, Cairns-Smith S, George BP, Palisch C, Dorsey ER. The anatomy of medical research: US and international comparisons. JAMA. 2015;313(2):174–89.
10. Campbell MJ. Medical statistics. Chester: Wiley; 1990. p. 393.
11. Greenfield ML, Kuhn JE, Wojtys EM. A statistics primer: descriptive measures for continuous data. Am J Sports Med. 1997;25(5):720–3.
12. Kuhn JE, Greenfield ML, Wojtys EM. A statistics primer. Prevalence, incidence, relative risks, and odds ratios: some epidemiologic concepts in the sports medicine literature. Am J Sports Med. 1997;25(3):414–6.

Chapter 16
Innovation for Surgeon Inventors

Stephen Bartol

Introduction

Every week surgeons come to me asking, "What do I do with my idea? How do I make money from this?" Perhaps even more often I get asked, "I am showing my invention to a medical device company next week. Do you think that is a good idea? I think they want to work with me but will they steal it? Would you mind taking a quick look and telling me what to do?"

This chapter is for surgeons who have these questions. It is not intended to be an all-inclusive guide to product commercialization nor is it intended to be an entrepreneur's handbook, but it will provide an overview of the topics that are most relevant to you as a surgeon inventor. It will help you ask the right questions, seek the right help, and map out a game plan for moving forward with your concept.

For most surgeons, coming up with new ideas is easy. Surgeons are constantly searching for better ways to do things. Whether it is looking for a faster, safer way to operate, a better surgical outcome, more efficient patient throughput, or improved patient satisfaction, continuous improvement has always been at the forefront of surgical practice.

Most of the ideas that come from surgeons involve either practice-based or mission-based initiatives: they help the surgeon improve their own practice or they help with the overall mission of providing better patient care. While these things are important, they usually have no real monetary value in the broader market. We certainly encourage surgeons to continue working on such ideas, improving patient care, and improving the bottom line for their practice, but it is not the intent of this chapter to deal with these noncommercial innovations. In this chapter, we will focus on the other type of innovations: those that do have market potential and which may

S. Bartol
CMO for Henry Ford Innovations, Henry Ford Health System, Department of Orthopedic Surgery, Detroit, MI, USA

E. C. Makhni et al. (eds.), *Orthopedic Practice Management*,
https://doi.org/10.1007/978-3-319-96938-1_16

be commercialized. We will review how to recognize a good idea, how to protect it, evaluate it, target a specific market, finance it, and pitch it.

Why Innovate?

We innovate for many reasons. Some do it because they like to create things; they enjoy the sense of satisfaction that comes from making something new. For those who are competitive, it may be a desire to be recognized for an accomplishment or to build a more lasting legacy. For most, there is a desire to improve things, to make the world a better place or more simply put, provide better patient care. At the end of the day, however, there is always one overlying motive that ultimately drives commercially viable innovation and determines success: making money.

To make money an invention must add value. When we ask, "Will this idea make money?" we are really asking, "Will people voluntarily give up something of value to get this?" Often, they will not, and the determining factor is "how much value does this product bring?"

When we talk about value, it is most important to understand how it is measured. On the surface, a product's value is how much someone will pay for it. But determining that is tricky. It depends on what motivates people. When I started my career in surgery some 25 years ago, surgeons placed great value on convenience and ease of use. If a product made a surgical technique easier to perform, surgeons would use it and hospitals would buy it for them to use, passing the cost on to insurers and patients who would pay for it. Those days are over. No one is paying much for surgeon convenience these days and that is because value is measured differently.

Every stakeholder in the product's lifecycle sees value differently. For surgeons, convenience, ease of use, and speed of surgery are very important. For patients, comfort, safety, and outcomes are paramount. For hospitals, it is all about market share and case margins, and for insurers it is all about global costs.

So who ultimately determines the value of a product? The answer depends on which of the stakeholders has the power to choose the product: who gets to make decisions. In 1992, the answer was clearly the surgeon. Surgeons ruled in those days and got to choose what was most important to them when choosing products. If an inventor came to market with a product that offered improved speed and reduced complications, successful adoption was almost a guarantee. Why does not that happen today? This is because power has shifted away from individual providers to large healthcare organizations and payers. The causes of that shift and the ramifications for surgeons are way beyond the scope of this chapter, but the effects are critical to understand if you are going to become a surgeon inventor in today's world.

Decisions about the use of products today, whether we are talking about implants, surgical tools, medications, or practice management tools, are largely made by hospitals, which are influenced most heavily by insurers and government payers. Recognizing that dynamic is critical to success as an inventor.

Cost is clearly a key factor in the adoption of innovative products in today's world. When looking at costs, the inventor needs to think of things in terms of value proposition for the stakeholder that holds the power to make decisions. If a product allows a surgeon to work faster, then that time must translate to the bottom line if the product is to be adopted. It is not enough to simply make a surgeon's work easier. If a product improves safety or provides better outcomes, then the savings through risk reduction must be calculated, and value judged accordingly. A product that reduces pain post-op or which speeds return to ADLs may seem valuable to a patient or a surgeon, but may be of no concern to the hospital or the payer. Does patient comfort lead to improved satisfaction and does that translate to better pay-for-performance payouts? Perhaps, but the value may be much less than the inventor is hoping. Does an earlier return to work matter to the payer? Probably not, but a decreased likelihood of readmission probably does. A shorter length of stay (LOS) may or may not be important to the payer, depending on the payment structure. If hospital payment is by DRG, then the hospital wants a reduced LOS but the payer does not care. Ultimately, it is possible to measure value from the perspective of the power stakeholder but to do so the surgeon inventor must have a clear understanding of the healthcare industry and the various stakeholders in it.

I have had many surgeons come to me in the last couple of years complaining that the age of innovation in surgery is over because surgeons no longer have the power to choose their own products. It is true that many implants have become commoditized, prices have plummeted, and great barriers have been erected to the introduction of new technology. It is also true that frontline healthcare providers have much less decision-making power than they once had. But, despite all this, the need for innovation is greater than ever.

The biggest driver of innovation in the world of healthcare is the aging population. Every day 10,000 baby boomers in America turn 65. Those over 65 will make up greater than 20% of the population by 2040 and 90% of those over 65 have a chronic disease of some sort. By 2040, healthcare spending in the USA will likely reach 26–30% of total GDP [1]. Demand for "better health" is growing at an alarming rate, and the opportunities for improving health through better products have never been greater. Yes, the market has changed and power has shifted, but the need for innovation is growing and greater than ever. Innovators simply need to adjust their way of viewing the market and adjust their value propositions accordingly.

As a surgeon inventor, you should not get lost in the healthcare delivery model. Remember that the key determinants of health include many things other than what we do as surgeons. Lifestyle, the environment, and genetics, all play a greater role in overall population health than healthcare delivery for the sick. Healthcare delivery makes up only about 10% of the overall spend on global health, and of healthcare dollars spent, 75% are spent on chronic disease management rather than acute care. Surgery and acute care delivery play relatively small roles in the global health market and finding value may be easier in other arenas. As an inventor, you should therefore think outside the *or*, that is, where most of the money is. As surgeons, sitting at the top of the health-provider food chain, we often forget that we have a unique perspective on population health and we share a level of understanding and expertise that is not trivial. Opportunities for innovation exist throughout the spectrum of global health determinants.

So, I encourage you to think beyond the *or* and think of the healthcare system as a whole when creating ideas. Think beyond how the product impacts the healthcare user and healthcare consumer. Think about all of the various stakeholders. There is a lot of value to be created but you need to find the right fit.

Intellectual Property

So, you have an idea. Maybe it is a new gadget that makes it safer to insert implants or maybe it is a tool that helps people stay healthier. Whatever the idea, you need to protect your intellectual property (IP) and in doing so create additional asset value.

There are several forms of IP. I like to think of IP broadly in these five categories:

- Patents
- Trade secrets
- Copyrights
- Trademarks
- Know-how

Each of these is designed to offer protection for ideas in some way and the two of greatest importance to surgeon inventors are patents and trade secrets.

Patents

A patent is a limited right to a monopoly that prevents anyone else from making, using, selling, or importing an invention for a defined period (usually 20 years). To be patentable, an idea must fulfill several criteria. It must be useful, novel, and non-obvious. It also must be truly invented by the inventor, it cannot be abandoned by the inventor, and it must not be publicly disclosed prior to the application.

Any number of things may be the subject matter of a patent. It may be a process (such as a method for synthesizing a product), a machine (such as a bone reamer), a manufactured product (a screw or a surgical tool), or a unique composition of matter (such as a new molecule).

Proving that your idea is novel begins with a patentability search. When searching you are looking for prior art in the form of prior patents, published patent applications, general publications, prior public use, or public knowledge. This search can be difficult, and it is essential that it be thorough. Even a single podium presentation or a publication in an obscure Russian journal can invalidate your patent by rendering it not novel. You can start the search process yourself, using either Google Patents or the United States Patent and Trademark Office (USPTO) website, but generally you will need to get professional help when moving beyond a preliminary search. I usually start with a search of US patents using Google Patents. I pick a few keywords related to the idea and read all the patents that come up. I am usually happy when I have read several hundred patents without finding anything like my claim(s). Next, I do a thorough literature review starting on PubMed. If nothing turns up in my search, then it is time to turn the project over to a patent attorney. The attorney will then have his search team complete the search in greater detail. They will continue the search of US patents and extend the literature search, digging through meeting presentations, technical databases, and non-US patents.

The purpose of the search is to determine that the idea is both novel and nonobvious. "Nonobvious" means that your idea is not simply an extension of a previous idea. Repurposing a tool for a new use is usually not patentable if that new application is obvious. Sometimes, it takes some argument to reach conclusions and a patent attorney can help you sort through whether your idea is both novel and nonobvious.

In medicine, there is often a tendency to spread ideas openly before they have been vetted for patentability. There is great pressure to publish and present research results early, especially in the academic community. Inventors need to resist that pressure if they want to patent their ideas. Public disclosure might include presenting the idea to one or several people or it may include public use. When you think of an idea, therefore, it is critical to document carefully and keep it quiet until a search for patentability is completed. Discussing it openly with your colleagues or sharing it in a podium presentation will invalidate its patentability. Before you present your research, talk to your patent attorney and let him know what you plan to disclose. It may be possible to talk about your research findings without disclosing the invention, and if not, you may want to file a provisional patent quickly.

Broadly speaking, there are two types of patents that you need to understand: provisional patents and utility patents. The provisional patent is essentially a holding place. The USPTO uses a "first-to-file" system for determining who has the right to patent. Filing a provisional patent places a time stamp on your idea and filing it protects you, allowing you time to further explore and develop the idea. The provisional patent buys a year, during which time the inventor can do further research, seek additional help in developing and testing ideas, and refine the patent claims.

Within a year of filing a provisional patent, a utility patent must be filed. If not, then the patent is abandoned and the ideas disclosed in the provisional patent become public domain and cannot be patented in the future. While a provisional patent may be somewhat vague in its content, the utility patent spells out the definitive claims of the patent.

Some surgeons balk at the cost of filing patents and ask me if they can do it on their own to save money. Experienced inventors may occasionally file a provisional application themselves but generally this is *not* recommended and only a fool files his own utility patent application. My advice to surgeon inventors is to spend their time more productively in the *or* making money to spend on a good patent attorney. It will be money well spent.

There are five key elements of a patent application: (1) data about the inventor(s), (2) the specification, (3) the claims, (4) the abstract, and (5) the drawings. To begin, it is essential to understand what constitutes inventorship. An inventor is a person who contributes to the claims of a patentable invention. The key is "contribution to a claim or claims." A person who made a physical embodiment of the invention may not be an inventor, no matter how difficult it was to reduce the invention to practice. The contribution must be to the idea, as spelled out in the claims. Someone who contributes labor or research, no matter how brilliant or hardworking, is not an inventor unless they contributed to at least one of the patent claims. When two or more persons make an invention jointly, they should apply for a patent jointly. They need not have worked physically together or at the same time, and they need not have contributed equally or to every claim in the patent. Inventorship simply means they contributed to at least one claim.

Getting it right is really important. Failure to list an inventor on a patent application can invalidate the patent since filing without an inventor's name could be seen as withholding key information from the Patent Office. Honest mistakes do happen and inventorship can be corrected, provided there was no deception intent, but getting it right at the outset will save a lot of grief. If in doubt, clarify it before filing.

Good records are critical in determining inventorship. Each inventor's contribution should be well documented. You cannot afford to have someone file evidence that invalidates a patent because his or her name was left off. If you have research assistants, students, residents, or employees working for you on a project, make it clear in advance whether their ideas contributed to a claim. If there is a dispute, I recommend meeting with the patent attorney and discussing openly who contributed what. The attorney can determine, often by reviewing records, whether inventorship should apply to an individual's contribution.

The patent document starts with an abstract, which is a precise summary of the invention disclosed. Although this is just a summary, it should be crafted with great care since courts will often rely on it to construe claims. It should be at least as broad as the broadest claim.

The patent specification, also called the disclosure, describes the invention in detail. It should include cross-references to related patents, a thorough background to aid in understanding the invention, detailed descriptions of drawings, and a detailed description of the invention. This description must include the ways and means to make and use the invention "in such full, clear, concise and exact terms as to enable one skilled in the art to which it pertains, or with which it is most nearly connected, to make and use" it. The specification also describes the inventors "contemplated" embodiments of the invention. All embodiments need not be known or disclosed in the patent, but a description of at least some embodiment greatly increases the chance that the patent will be granted.

The specific claims are the core of a patent and appear at the end of the document. They define the limits of exactly what the patent does and does not cover. My advice to surgeon inventors is: "Do not write claims yourself." Understand them, but get help from an experienced patent attorney in writing them. These are the heart and soul of the patent. The patentee has the right to exclude others from making, using, or selling only those things that are described by the claims.

A patent grants the inventor or assignee the exclusive right to commercialization for a limited period of time. *All* listed inventors have this right, regardless of how much they individually contributed to the patent. It is important therefore that the patent be assigned to a single entity at the time of application. A patent with more than one inventor has *limited value* without an assignee. Discuss this with your attorney if you do not understand it, but do not ignore it. Your attorney will generally recommend that all inventors form an entity (such as an LLC or a corporation) and assign their rights to it. The ownership of the entity (and hence the ownership of the patent) can then be sold or divided, according to whatever formula the inventors decide upon. Usually, ownership will be divided by degree of contribution.

Trade Secrets

When a patent is granted, the patent rights are granted in exchange for public disclosure. In other words, you are giving up your secrets in exchange for a time-limited monopoly. There are many instances where this is not wise. Some things are best kept secret. A trade secret is any confidential (nonpublic) information, including formulas, algorithms, manufacturing and fabrication techniques, business plans, supplier lists, costs, plans, etc. The advantage of a trade secret is that its lifespan is infinite, or as long as it remains a secret. Perhaps, the best example of a trade secret is the Coke formula. No one outside of a select few at Coca-Cola knows what the formula is. It has never been patented. If it had, it would be available for all to read and copy. Instead of patenting it, the founders elected to keep it a secret, and, in doing so, added tremendous value to their product.

No registration is required to establish a trade secret. Careful consideration should be given to whether a patent is filed or the idea kept secret. If you are confident that the secret can be kept, that the product can *never* be reverse engineered, and that the product lifecycle may exceed 20 years, then keeping a trade secret may be a preferred option. As always, discuss this with your IP attorney before making a final decision.

IP Ownership

For many surgeons, employed practice is becoming the norm rather than the exception. This can be problematic when it comes to ownership of intellectual property. Most healthcare institutions and academic centers have strict policies that require employees to assign all inventions to the employer. There may or may not be an agreement to share the financial rewards with the inventors. *You need to clarify this before you sign a contract of employment*. I cannot overemphasize this. The most common problem that surgeon inventors bring to me is the problem of employment contracts that limit or prevent the inventor's ability to make money from their inventions. This must be thought about and resolved before, rather than after, the fact.

If you have not yet signed a contract, this issue needs to be put on the table and discussed prior to any hire. If you already have an employment contract in place, get it out and read the IP clause carefully. If you do not see an IP clause, you are not necessarily off the hook. In many jurisdictions, an employer will own the rights to work for hire, which means that intellectual property created during the course of employment probably belongs to the employer. Sticking your head in the sand and ignoring this is not a strategy. Trying to hide the invention or secretly sell it will NOT work. When it comes time to sell a license to the invention or to raise money from investors to develop it, no one will pay you a dime until a full release is obtained from your employer. So, your employer is going to find out. You will need to get a signed release document. You may as well clarify things up front. This topic is much too big to cover in detail in this chapter but I want to emphasize the need to get legal advice and get it early. Discuss things early on with your own (not your employer's) attorney, preferably before you take any job working for someone else.

Understanding, Choosing, and Evaluating Your Market

Before spending money developing prototypes, you first must determine if you have an idea that is worth spending your money on. The first thing to do is to match your product to a specific market need. In their book *Biodesign: The Process of Innovating Medical Technologies* [2], the authors put forth the key premise that innovation is a process: a skill that can be learned. The process is simple in form: first identify, then invent, and finally implement. I strongly recommend the book to those who are interested in creating or improving medical devices. In practice, most of the surgeons who come to me with ideas have already "invented" something and then need to work backward to determine just what problem they are solving and who they are solving it for.

As we discussed earlier in this chapter, there is a market dynamic that must be recognized. Every stakeholder has a different viewpoint and therefore different needs. Not every stakeholder has the same degree of decision-making power or influence. Moreover, the dynamic is constantly changing. Determining whose need you want to target is very dependent on market acceptance. We will discuss adoption in more detail later in this chapter, but it must be considered at the earliest stage of idea/product development. There is little to be gained from developing an idea that meets the needs of a low priority stakeholder. Meeting a critical need for a stakeholder who holds all the cards is a different matter altogether. The follow-up to this is market size consideration. If a complex procedure using your device can be performed by only a select group of extremely talented academic surgeons, few of whom experience difficulties, you probably should not bother developing your idea, since the market is just too small. Meeting an overwhelming need experienced by all surgeons in the community setting is another matter altogether.

There is no perfect way to define a need. Sometimes, a need is identified through personal experience. This is common among surgeons. You feel the frustration of a problem in the OR and you attempt to solve it. The good thing about this is that the problem is immediately "validated." It is real, because you experienced it. On the con side, it probably involves very "in the box" thinking, may not be so novel, and it may not be scalable in the market (you might be the only person who experiences this problem).

An alternative way to approach the market is to survey or otherwise engage potential customers. This can be a good approach because it is quantifiable and it can be very iterative, with ideas building on each another. On the con side are cost and access. Getting access to a good representation of the market may be challenging. When surveying potential customers, you should be careful who you ask. If you approach only "experts" in the field, you probably will not get a good idea of the problems experienced by "average" users. You also should be careful what you ask. I never ask potential customers what they want. They usually do not know. Henry Ford once famously said, "If I had asked people what they wanted, they would have said: 'faster horses'." Asking customers what they want will confine the inventor to boxes. Remember, there are no boxes. What you want to know is what is "causing pain" for the customer and how many potential customers are feeling that pain.

Perhaps, the best method to learn whether your idea meets a need is to learn lessons by failing fast. Unfortunately, this is not always applicable and may be tough in a regulated industry like healthcare. It is not impossible, however, and I have often done a quick trial of an idea in an animal lab, subsequently saving a fortune in development costs by proving or disproving a concept quickly.

Quantitative Analysis

Once you have found a market opportunity and found a solution to meet it, the next step requires you to do some math and quantify that opportunity. The first step in quantifying things is to develop a business model: a description of how you make money. Business plans are not all that helpful at this stage so do not waste your time. A business model that works for your idea is essential, however. Nothing in business works unless you have something to sell and a way to make money doing it. Surprisingly, many inventors come with prototypes already developed without having figured out how they will make money. Think about this before you spend time and money on product development or testing. The questions to ask yourself are not hard. Will you sell capital or consumables? Perhaps, it is both or perhaps you give away capital to attract sales of disposables. Is a contract, license, or subscription model the right option for you? Any of these choices could work for different products in different markets. A little brainstorming will tell you which options are open to you. Some market research and number crunching will quickly tell you which are the most viable choices for your idea.

Once you have a business model, a financial model is needed before a decision can be made about investing money. Fundamentally, the financial model is a time-phased comparison of proceeds to costs. My experience with many surgeon inventors is that they want to bow out at this stage, either because they do not understand the premise or because they are afraid of the financial risk taking and do not want to deal with it. My advice is get some help and press on. As with the IP issues discussed earlier, a little professional help can save you a lot of time and money.

Building a financial model is not much different from developing a budget for your household or your practice; it is just bigger in scope and contains a lot more uncertainty. All sources of income (grants, investments, sales, etc.) and all sources of expenses (operating costs, interest, taxes, legal, etc.) are considered. Since you have not built the business yet, some assumptions are needed to estimate these numbers. Make notes of what your assumptions are. Your investors will want to know what assumptions you made and why you did so. Good input leads to good output so a sound understanding of the project and the market are needed. As a surgeon, you likely have a very solid understanding of what is happening in healthcare and what is likely to happen in the future and your inputs will be valuable in making the modeling assumptions.

The most important thing to remember when building a financial model is that cash is king. Debt is paid out of cash flow, not net worth, so cash flow is of paramount importance. Even if net worth is growing, the plan will fail if you run out of cash. At the end of the day, economic modeling allows one to discern cash flow and align decision-making accordingly.

There are a few basic cautions that should be applied to financial modeling. The first is this: all models are wrong (though useful). Since the numbers in a model are "made up" based on assumptions, they are bound to be wrong. Good input increases the probability that the numbers are close, and iterative review will enhance accuracy as time goes on.

Second, opportunity cost does not weigh in on calculations in the financial model. They must be considered separately. When someone invests in your project, they are giving up an opportunity to make money elsewhere. That lost opportunity constitutes their "hurdle" to investment. Similarly, if you as a surgeon spend time on inventing products or building a company, you are giving up income earned in your practice. Those are your opportunity costs. Potential gains in the financial model must be weighed against your opportunity losses.

That brings us an important point that is often difficult for many surgeons to grasp. As a surgeon, you attach a certain value to your time. It is probably several hundred dollars an hour for most of the things you do. You may even get paid periodically by device manufacturers to help with product validation or testing. They likely pay you several hundred dollars an hour for your time. Some surgeons, new to innovation, will try to add their time to a financial model, paying themselves several hundred dollars an hour for that time. Your time as an inventor or product developer is not worth the same as it is as a surgeon. The time that you as the inventor put into your idea is basically worth zero dollars. The value of the idea must stand for itself. Whether you will ultimately see a return on investment (ROI) is based on a simple formula: add your out of pocket expenses and subtract that total from your net proceeds. If the number is bigger than your opportunity losses, then you have a positive ROI. When surgeon inventors approach an investor and say their patent is worth 2 million dollars because they spent 2 years working on it, it tells me they do not understand the fundamentals. Do not make that mistake. An idea drawn on a napkin is generally worth the price of a used napkin. Your time as an inventor is worth even less. Your idea is only worth something if it will lead to a significantly positive ROI. Your job as the inventor is to increase the asset value of your idea by adding value to it. You add value with IP protection, a favorable market validation, working prototypes, demonstrated first human use, regulatory approval, positive outcomes form independent clinical studies, and sales. Your financial plan must show how you are adding asset value and in the end, it must demonstrate a satisfactory ROI.

The financial model is therefore a very important document. It is a living document; constantly changing as new and better information becomes available. It may start as simply a feasibility study to determine if you really have something, but as money is invested, it needs to evolve into a thorough analysis of the product and its potential in the market. Your credibility as an inventor will depend in great part on what is in this document and how well you can defend what it says. My advice, therefore, is get help in preparing your financial model, be conservative in your estimates, and be prepared to defend all the assumptions made in the calculations.

Financing Your Project

Once you have a financial model, the next concern is finding the money to make it happen. It is important to remember that value creation is not a linear process. The objective is to grow value in a stepwise fashion as resources (time and money) are added. (Fig. 16.1) Good planning is needed to determine how much financing is required to reach the next step in value creation. Clearly, inadequate funding means the project will fail and money will be lost. It is just as concerning when excess funding is put into place. Raising money that is not yet needed simply dilutes share value and fails to yield expected returns for the investors. As shown in Fig. 16.1, the slope of the growth curve in each segment is the critical factor. It must match the anticipated rate of return for the investor.

A good financing strategy answers important questions. First, it defines how much money is needed in total. The answer lies in the financial model. Good research, sound knowledge of the market, and iterative improvements as time goes on all improve accuracy of that model. The second question to ask is how many tranches are needed. An individual tranche should allow the developers to achieve the next milestone in value creation. Timing of fundraising is important so that momentum is not lost. Since you will spend roughly 10 times as much time raising

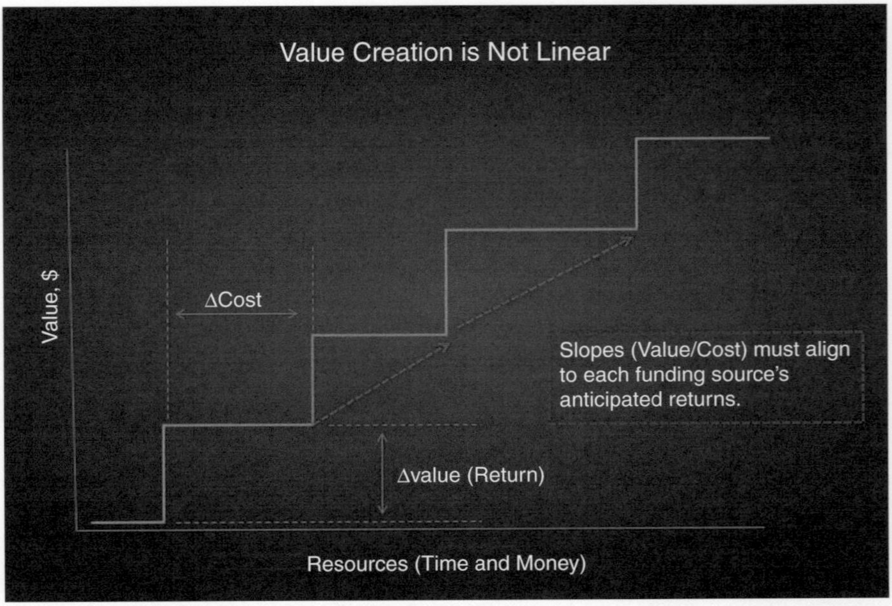

Fig. 16.1 Value creation

money as you do on actual value creation, you need to think ahead and time each raise.

Where do you get the money to develop your idea? There are many sources, some more expensive than others. Money out of your own pocket is not "free." It comes with real as well as opportunity costs that must be considered. You will need to put money into your own project, however, since investors are going to want to see that you have something at stake. Investing only your time is not acceptable in most cases. Remember, your time is not worth much, but your hard-earned dollars are. Do not make the mistake of going to investors looking for cash if you have not shown that you believe in your own project by putting your own money into it.

There are some "free" sources of capital that you may want to explore. These come in the form of grants, and examples are the NIH Small Business Innovation Research (SBIR) and Small Business Technology Transfer (STTR) programs. There are others that you should watch for, usually designed to stimulate a specific aspect of the economy, or to explore specific needs identified by the government. Whether you should take advantage of these programs is a strategic decision that you will have to consider carefully. Grants are based on bare bones budgets and will not provide money for commercialization, so while they can supplement, they cannot form a funding strategy by themselves. It also takes time to write grant applications. Generally, a lot of time. You will need to weigh the opportunity cost. Typically, my advice to inventors is to use grants when they will not risk lost momentum. Driving the project forward as quickly as possible is the primary objective and if a grant will slow you down, do not waste your time. It is probably "cheaper" to get money elsewhere. If you do decide to "go for" a grant, hire some help to write the application. There are usually lots of unemployed PhDs around who are better at grant writing than you.

Another source for capital often sought by surgeon inventors is strategic partners. As a surgeon, you probably already know who they are. They are the companies who might be interested in your idea. These organizations are good sources of funds because their interest has a huge validation effect. Other investors will be attracted by the fact that a strategic partner has indicated an interest. There are major drawbacks, however. Strategic partners often demand onerous milestones and big companies often will not tolerate the ups and downs and general uncertainty that you are likely to experience early on. While having a strategic partner may take some of the funding pressure off, you may be better off in the end by remaining neutral, especially during those early growing pains. If you do sign on with a strategic, they will often look for distribution rights in return. While this may be a good way to tackle distribution problem, you should consider very carefully what sort of effort is likely to be generated by their sales force. Many new products die in the bags of a salesforce that is not trained or adequately motivated to sell a new product.

Most often inventors start with money from their own pocket followed by funds from friends and family. Taking money from friends and family can be risky both ways. On the one hand, if you do not take their money and you end up making a fortune, they may be upset. On the other hand, the more likely scenario is that you take their money and lose it all. They may be prepared to forgive you but you may not forgive yourself. I have two basic guidelines for inventors considering taking money from friends and family. First, only take money from those who are accredited or qualified investors. To those that are not, you simply say that the rules do not allow you to take their money. If you do not understand these terms, talk to your attorney before you raise any money. Second, when taking money from friends and family, only allow them to invest money they can afford to lose, that is, usually 5–10% of their non-retirement investment portfolio. Never, ever allow anyone to invest retirement money in your ideas. And never, ever allow anyone, including yourself, to mortgage his or her home for your invention.

Perhaps, the best source of funds, and certainly one that you will want to nurture relationships with if you are going to be a serial inventor, is angels. Angels are wealthy individuals who play in the high-risk funding world. Often, they are entrepreneurs who started like you, were successful in "making it" themselves, and are now using their newfound wealth to stay in the game. Typically, they want to stay involved somehow, often as advisors, and very often they have some specific industry knowledge or expertise. This can prove very helpful but can be deadly too, so tread carefully. Angels typically invest smaller amounts than VC and will often organize into groups to pool funds and mitigate risk. Generally, they tend to stay local and focus on industries that they know and understand. They also want to know you well and will typically spend a lot of time getting to know a project and the people behind it. I have always thought of my angel investors as "partners" in the business and I choose my partners very, very carefully. Angels will often play where institutional investors fear to tread and they tend to be much more patient than the venture capital (VC) funds, so the right angel can be an excellent partner to have.

Institutional venture capital (VC) funds are professionally managed funds that invest in early-stage companies. Typically, they will have target investment allotments ($2–5 M, Series A) with the intent of follow-on investment in future tranches. They only invest in areas where they have experience and can add value. Often seen as "evil," their terms are usually very dilutive and can be somewhat overbearing, usually demanding control. Once that happens, technology is no longer the focus, the founder's vision eliminated, and attention directed at meeting expected returns within a specific timeframe. The good news about VC funds is that if they want to invest in you, then you must have a big idea. If you are approaching institutions for money, my advice is to get help the first time you do this. The stakes are very high when dealing with these professionals, so get the professional help you need to negotiate the right deal for you.

Prototyping and Testing

Prototyping a new product should be done with specific objectives in mind. Do not run out to the nearest machine shop and spend your hard-earned money without a plan. Before you do that, start with the basics. Define the problem and assess the market opportunity. Good inventors spend far more time defining the problem than they spend on the solution. Too often inventors rush to prototype, only to discover that they need to scrap their design and start all over again because the prototype does not solve their target market's problem. Understanding the problem better will allow you to brainstorm multiple viable solutions and choose the best one. The earlier you make good choices, the faster and cheaper it will be to get to market. It is far cheaper to fix things early through proper planning than to try and change things later when you are close to market.

Before you spend any money, you need a critical analysis of your financial plan. That means you need to accept criticism of your idea and you need to be able to reject ideas that are not financially viable. Good inventors save themselves a lot of money and a lot of grief by killing most of their ideas long before they ever build a prototype. If the numbers do not work, then the prototype will not save you. Kill the project.

Too often surgeon inventors fail to take time for adequate supporting documentation. Documentation is essential for good IP protection of course but it is also essential in preparing for regulatory submissions and planning quality manufacturing. Plowing ahead without proper planning and documentation is a big mistake because it means that you will need to backtrack and repeat much of what you have already done just to satisfy quality manufacturing and regulatory requirements. Get help with this. Careful documentation is not something that comes naturally to surgeons who are used to just fixing things. I recommend that you work closely with a skilled engineer or engineering team who are experienced with medical device development. They will save you a lot of time and money in the end. Documentation and independent validation are essential at every stage, so make sure that it is getting written down.

Regulatory Basics

Getting a product to market is expensive, especially in healthcare where regulatory controls are stringent. Stanford University prepared a report in 2010 titled *FDA Impact on US Medical Technology Innovation: A survey of Over 200 Medical technology Companies* [3]. The study was designed to address the need for data used to evaluate the impact of US medical device regulation on innovation and patients. The study showed that the average cost of taking a medical device from conception through clearance is $31 M for 510(k) products and $91 M if a PMA is required. These are staggering numbers and enough to discourage most inventors from even considering getting their own regulatory clearance or approval. As with other aspects of the innovation process, my advice is to get help. Having the FDA stamp adds tremendous asset value so if possible, get help, press on, and tackle the regulatory hurdle.

The FDA cares about two things: safety and efficacy. "Value" and "comparative effectiveness," while critical for marketing your product, are of no concern to the FDA. Since most of the innovations that surgeons will develop fall into the device category, I will limit my discussion here to devices. While the protocols for devices are simpler than those for drugs, the process is much more complex in terms of knowing how to approach the FDA.

Devices are viewed according to their safety profile. Each is placed in a class. Class 1 devices are low-risk devices that by themselves pose no inherent safety risk. They include most common surgical dissection instruments and tools such as scalpels, retractors, bone elevators, and chisels. Class 2 devices carry greater safety risk and include most of our orthopedic implants and many of the tools used to measure or monitor what we as surgeons do. Class 3 devices are those devices that deal with life-threatening matters. Heart valves and lasers are good examples.

Much of the confusion and argument around FDA classification of devices concerns Class 2 devices and whether a premarket "approval" (PMA) is required. A PMA means that clinical study is required to demonstrate safety and efficacy. This is both time-consuming and extremely expensive. A device that requires a PMA, therefore, has a much higher hurdle to achieve a satisfactory ROI. An exemption to a PMA is given to certain Class 2 devices. Section 510(k) of the Act allows the FDA to "clear" devices without a PMA if the device is "substantially equivalent" to another device that is already approved. The new device must be "at least" as safe and effective as the predicate device. You should be aware that there is an imbalance between the FDA and Patent Office conversations, but this is not necessarily a contradiction. While you want to demonstrate to the USPTO that your device is "novel and nonobvious," you want to convince the FDA that there is "substantial equivalency" to a predicate device with respect to safety and efficacy.

The surgeon inventor can play a vital role in the regulatory process by helping to prepare documents for submission. Time costs money, so speed is of the essence, and an experienced regulatory consultant can save you a tremendous amount of time. Work closely with your consultants. To move quickly through the FDA, your application must be clearly understood. Indications for use need to be specific and clear. It is your job as the surgeon inventor to explain these indications. The wording is critical because future marketing of the device is limited to the wording that is "cleared." The instructions for use are particularly important as well and must be simply and clearly stated so that even a nonmedical person can understand them. Remember that safety is of paramount importance and attention to safety details must be evident in the document.

The people working at the FDA are, for the most part, less well trained and far less experienced in your field than you are. As with everything else you do in business, relationships matter. In my experience, the people at the FDA, for the most part, want to be helpful. Write the submission, therefore, as a document that speaks for itself, does not assume a vast knowledge base, and delivers a clear message. Make sure it is complete. Communicate openly and frequently. Like many government employees, FDA workers are often overworked, with a massive pile of documents on their desk that seems to grow daily. Your submission first goes to an "Acceptance Review." If it is incomplete, it will be rejected from acceptance and you need to respond quickly to fill in deficiencies. The lead reviewer may choose to continue with an "interactive review" in which case they will contact you by email or phone. Respond immediately and be helpful. Pool together whatever resources are needed and answer their questions quickly and completely. Delays are costly so do not let your submission drift to the bottom of the pile.

There is an alternative pathway for expedited approval called a Humanitarian Device Exemption (HDE). This applies to very few commercially viable devices. A Humanitarian Use Device is one used to treat rare conditions that affect <4000 people in the USA annually. Use of an HUD requires local IRB approval and supervision, and the applicant must demonstrate that there are no comparable devices available to treat or diagnose the disease or condition, and that they could otherwise not bring the device to market.

Adoption

After you have invented your product, successfully obtained IP protection, financed, development, prototyped, tested, and cleared regulatory hurdles, you meet the most difficult challenge in Healthcare Innovation: gaining adoption. New inventors often make a big mistake and assume that their idea is so brilliant that the world will beat a path to their door. Let me assure you, it never happens.

Marketing products is a complex subject, and I am certainly not able to deal with the entire topic in this chapter. I will discuss the two factors that are most important for surgeon inventors to understand: competition and reimbursement.

Inexperienced inventors often think their invention is so novel that there is no competition. Wrong. There is *always* competition. If you believe there is not, then you do not understand the market. Even if your product is a completely disruptive, brand new technology, it competes with something. Those who benefit from what the market is already doing are your competitors and they will fight you. Prepare yourself by understanding them. Know their strengths and weakness and ready yourself for battle.

Naïve, first-time inventors often believe that they will capture market share quickly and they build financial models that reflect unrealistically rapid growth. Do not make the mistake of thinking that you will capture 25% market share in 3 years just because your technology is better. Look at top industries and see what the market share of leaders is on average. It is around 20% for most industries. Look at the medical device sector that you are entering. You will find that leaders typically have between 5% and 30% of the market. Do not assume that competitors will roll over and let you beat them at their own game. They will not. You are going to work hard to get low single-digit percentages of the market. Plan accordingly.

First-time inventors also often make the mistake of assuming that competitors will gladly buy their IP and discard current products in favor of a new one, just because it is better. Again, this is wrong. Imagine the cost of doing that. Killing one product to replace it with another does not make business sense unless it leads to higher profits at the end of the day. If you want a large device company to buy or license your product, you need to understand how they make money and how you propose to add value for them. This takes us back to market need and the importance of understanding the market before you approach it with your product.

In the same way that there is this switching cost for device companies, there is always a switching cost for the consumer. It may be that there is a learning curve for your product. Learning curves result in increased risks, poorer outcomes, and lost time until the user becomes very familiar with your product. There may be costs that are already sunk into existing products or there may be contracts with existing suppliers that must be discarded. It may be that your new technology costs more to purchase or there may be implementation costs and training costs. It may simply be that the customer is a best friend of your competitor's salesmen and risks losing that relationship if they buy your product. Whatever the case, you should carefully consider what the customer must give up when they buy your product instead of whatever they are doing now. Those costs are barriers to your product. The better you understand them and prepare yourself to face them, the more likely your success.

Probably, the greatest barrier to adoption of products in healthcare is a mismatched reimbursement model. A lot of great products die because no one bothered to consider whether anyone would be paid for using them. End users in healthcare are usually healthcare providers, and the benefactors of products are usually patients.

Yet, neither of these stakeholders typically pays for a healthcare product. It is not enough to be cost-effective or result in better outcomes in American healthcare. If the product does not fit the current reimbursement landscape, then no one will use it.

I am often surprised by how few people in healthcare understand how the money flows. You need to think this through very carefully. Who is paying whom? How are providers paid? How does your product fit in? If decision-makers see increased costs as a result of using your product, then they will actively fight against it, even if it means that the system as a whole benefits from its use. As a surgeon, you can help plan by understanding reimbursement codes and reimbursement models well in advance, even before you build your business model. Failure to do so may mean that you meet an insurmountable barrier to adoption, sending you back to the drawing board.

The Pitch

Pitching your product or idea is an art. It is an art that can be learned through practice. I strongly recommend that you start by watching and learning from others who are good at this. I also strongly recommend that you enter business plan competitions or at least attend a few to learn from others.

We all have our individual strengths and not everyone is meant to be a pitch artist. As a surgeon inventor you probably, more than anyone, understand the problem you are solving and have the passion needed to drive the solution forward. If you find that you are not a natural at pitching, however, then as with everything else, get help. If you do allow someone else to give the pitch, just make sure that your understanding of the market and your passion to solve the market problem come through in what they say.

There are three pitches that you need to prepare: a 30-s elevator pitch, a 3-min quick pitch, and a 10-min full pitch. The hardest to develop is the shortest pitch. If you struggle with it, then you need to spend more time studying the problem and the market. In 30 s, you should be able to make someone understand the problem you are solving and how you are solving it. Tell that with passion and they will want to learn more.

While the 30-s pitch is all about getting your audience's attention, the 3-min pitch is about keeping them hooked. I suggest you focus on telling a story. Describe (quickly) the pain in the market. Then tell how your technology solves the problem. Say who your competitors are and why you are better, and then describe how you are going to make money. Do *not* spend time explaining your technology. You will lose your audience. Wait for them to ask questions. The goal of this pitch is to stimulate questions.

The ultimate pitch is the one that is usually reserved for a planned audience, a group of angel investors, for example. Usually, you will be given 10 min. Take 8 and end early, leaving more time for questions. *Never* go over. A good 10-min

Table 16.1 Common formula for the 10-min pitch

The pitch deck
Introduction
Need/value proposition
Technology/product
Market
Competition
Path to market and exit
Team
Next steps/use of funds
Financial information
Conclusion

pitch takes 8 min to deliver and leads to a 2-h discussion. Remember, investors invest in people, and your goal in the 10-min pitch is to *sell yourself*, not your technology.

There is a common formula to the 10-min pitch that you should generally follow (Table 16.1). First, introduce yourself (and your Company if you have one) and then explain the market need. Try to do this in a way that demonstrates your knowledge of value propositions. What is the problem you will address? This part should take no more than 30 s.

Next, tell how you solved the problem. Explain the product *briefly*. Do not go too heavily into the technology. You will lose your audience!

Move on to the market. Who are the customers? How big is the market? In this part, you must show that you know your market well and if the market is growing, tell them how. Know the numbers! If you do not know the market numbers, the audience will stop listening.

The competition comes next. Say who they are and tell why your product is better. You will again lose your audience with too much detail about technology so do not get hung up on that. Let the audience ask questions later. Your job in this section is to demonstrate that you know the competition and are prepared to fight them with a better solution.

The next step is to describe the path to market. This is where young entrepreneurs typically get lost. You must show that you know how to put money to work, develop, and deploy the product, leading ultimately to an exit. This step explains the business model and the business strategy and must show a solid understanding of the business.

Next, you should introduce the team. You cannot do this alone and you need to show that you understand that. Explain who is on your team and why they are qualified. If you have assembled an advisory board, introduce them too. It will show that you are willing to listen and learn from others.

Outline the "next steps" clearly. If you are asking for money, tell your audience how you will spend it. Show them your 12–24-month targets for development and commercialization.

Finally, comes the money. This is a (very) summarized version of your financial plan. Show how much money you need. Explain who the current investors/owners are and always end with the promise of making money.

When you conclude, wrap up quickly so that you can move on to questions. Name the product and provide the contact point going forward.

As you present this pitch, remember that it must tell a story. It is a story about a problem in the market and how you are solving that problem. Present the story with passion and leave your audience wanting to know more about you and your idea.

Final Thoughts

Fostering innovation in healthcare is no small feat. In this chapter, I have talked a lot about market needs and it has long been said that necessity is the mother of invention. That is certainly true. Fulfilling market needs is the single most important feature of great products. The challenge is finding the time, resources, and talent needed to recognize those market needs. Dzau et al. studied innovation in academic medical centers and concluded that innovation must be actively cultivated by teaching it, creating "space" for and supporting it, and providing opportunities for its implementation [4]. In other words, it takes dedicated time and financial support to be innovative. Innovation cannot be relegated to second-class status by the urgency of day-to-day operations, patient care, and the requirements of traditional research [4]. Ellner et al. also studied this and concluded that to be successful in academic medical centers, innovation programs must include robust funding for career development, curricula to develop skills, and new pathways for innovators to disseminate their work [5].

These challenges are even greater in private practice, where time is money and finding time to be creative seems all but impossible. The opportunity costs in private practice are huge. Every minute set aside for innovation is a lost opportunity for practice revenue. But if you want to create, you must make the time and take the time to do so. Without free time to be creative and to nurture ideas, innovation simply does not happen. Start by taking time to be by yourself. Sit in a boat fishing, read a novel, paint a picture, ride a bike, or go for a long run. Whatever works for you, do it. You need to be alone with your thoughts, away from the day-to-day distractions of patient care if you want to create. Next, establish a place where you and like-minded people can get together to brainstorm. Coffee shops and bars come to mind. Get out of the surgeons' lounge and get away from day-to-day work. Finally, establish a network of support people, focusing on people whose strengths are different from your own. Build a network around you that includes engineers, designers, patent attorneys, business consultants, and business advisors, and make sure that you take time to nurture and continuously grow that network.

Lastly, remember that as with everything else, you learn innovation by doing. You will likely fail in your first few attempts. This is hard for surgeons to accept because most surgeons have never failed at anything. You should recognize that 19 out of every 20 inventions are destined to fail and view each innovation failure as just another opportunity to learn how to do things better next time. Investors are going to want to see that you are experienced, so do not shy away from failure. Simply look for problems that cannot be solved, and put your skill and expertise to work and try to solve them. Awareness of the barriers you need to overcome will not guarantee you success in your enterprise, but knowledge of the various steps and the hurdles you must overcome will at least allow you to mitigate some of the inherent risks and help you increase your chance of success.

References

1. Fuchs VR. The gross domestic product and health care spending. N Engl J Med. 2013;369:107–9.
2. Yock PG, Zenios S, Makower J, Brinton TJ, Kumar UN, et al. Biodesign: the process of innovating medical technologies. 2nd ed: United Kingdom: Cambridge University Press; 2015.
3. FDA Impact on US Medical Technology Innovation: a survey of over 200 Medical Technology Companies. Advanced Medical Technology Association (AdvaMed); 2010.
4. Dzau VJ, Yoediono Z, Ellaissi WF, Cho AH. Fostering innovation in medicine and health care: what must academic health centers do? Acad Med. 2013;88(10):1424–9.
5. Ellner AL, Stout S, Sullivan EE, Griffiths EP, Mountjoy A, Phillips RS. Health systems innovation at academic health centers: leading in a new era of health care delivery. Acad Med. 2015;90(7):87280.

Index

E. C. Makhni et al. (eds.), *Orthopedic Practice Management*,
https://doi.org/10.1007/978-3-319-96938-1

C

D

MIX
Papier aus verantwortungsvollen Quellen
Paper from responsible sources
FSC® C105338

If you have any concerns about our products,
you can contact us on
ProductSafety@springernature.com

In case Publisher is established outside the EU,
the EU authorized representative is:
Springer Nature Customer Service Center GmbH
Europaplatz 3, 69115 Heidelberg, Germany

Printed by Libri Plureos GmbH
in Hamburg, Germany